Lippincott's Pathophysiology Series

RENAL PATHOPHYSIOLOGY

James A. Shayman, MD
Associate Professor of Medicine
Department of Internal Medicine
Division of Nephrology
University of Michigan Medical School
Ann Arbor, Michigan

With 6 contributing authors

J. B. Lippincott Company
Philadelphia

Acquisitions Editor: Richard Winters
Sponsoring Editor: Melissa James
Production Editor: Virginia Barishek
Interior Designer: Larry Pezzato
Cover Designer: Larry Pezzato
Indexer: L. Pilar Wyman
Production: P. M. Gordon Associates
Compositor: Pine Tree Composition
Printer/Binder: Courier Book Company/Kendallville
Cover Printer: Lehigh Press Lithographers

6   5   4   3   2   1

Library of Congress Cataloging-in-Publication Data

Renal pathophysiology / [edited by] James A. Shayman, with 6
    contributing authors.
        p.   cm. — (Lippincott's pathophysiology series)
    Includes bibliographical references and index.
    ISBN 0–397–51372–0 (alk. paper)
    1. Kidneys—Pathophysiology.   I. Shayman, James A.   II. Series.
    [DNLM: 1. Kidney—physiopathology.   WJ 301 R39343 1995]
RC903.9.R478   1995
616.6′107—dc20
DNLM/DLC
for Library of Congress   95–10443
                                                                      CIP

♾ This paper meets the requirements of ANSI/NISO Z39.48–1992 (Permanence of Paper).

The authors and publisher have exerted every effort to ensure that drug selection and dosage set forth in this text are in accord with current recommendations and practice at the time of publication. However, in view of ongoing research, changes in government regulations, and the constant flow of information relating to drug therapy and drug reactions, the reader is urged to check the package insert for each drug for any change in indications and dosage and for added warnings and precautions. This is particularly important when the recommended agent is a new or infrequently employed drug.

Lippincott's Pathophysiology Series

RENAL PATHOPHYSIOLOGY

In memory of my father,

Benjamin Shayman,

my first and best mentor

CONTRIBUTORS

Frank C. Brosius, MD

Assistant Professor of Medicine
Department of Internal Medicine
Division of Nephrology
University of Michigan Medical School
Ann Arbor, Michigan

H. David Humes, MD

Professor of Medicine
Department of Internal Medicine
Division of Nephrology
University of Michigan Medical School
Ann Arbor, Michigan

David Kershaw, MD

Lecturer in Pediatrics
Department of Pediatrics and Commu-
  nicable Diseases
Division of Pediatric Nephrology
University of Michigan Medical School
Ann Arbor, Michigan

James A. Shayman, MD

Associate Professor of Medicine
Department of Internal Medicine
Division of Nephrology
University of Michigan Medical School
Ann Arbor, Michigan

William E. Smoyer, MD

Assistant Professor of Pediatrics
Department of Pediatrics and Commu-
  nicable Diseases
Division of Pediatric Nephrology
University of Michigan Medical School
Ann Arbor, Michigan

Roger C. Wiggins, MD

Professor of Medicine
Department of Internal Medicine
Division of Nephrology
University of Michigan Medical School
Ann Arbor, Michigan

Eric W. Young, MD

Assistant Professor of Medicine
Department of Internal Medicine
Division of Nephrology
University of Michigan Medical School
Ann Arbor, Michigan

PREFACE

*I*n 1992, the Dean of the University of Michigan Medical School directed the faculty to restructure the medical school curriculum. In reviewing the materials available for the second-year course on renal pathophysiology, we concluded that there was no ideal text for second-year medical students. Although several excellent pathophysiology texts are available, in general, these tend to be too long and too detailed to be easily mastered within a 2-week course. As a result, many students forego reading a text to concentrate on class notes and handouts. Unfortunately, this often results in an inadequate comprehension of fundamental renal pathophysiology. This book was written in an attempt to rectify this problem.

An ideal text should be concise and cogent. It should be sufficiently challenging to hold the interest of the brightest students. Ideally, the text should also prepare the student to begin his or her clinical rotations with a fundamental sense of how to approach a patient with an electrolyte or renal abnormality and an understanding of the principles underlying common diagnostics and therapeutics. Although this text is far from ideal, it was written with these goals in mind.

Renal Pathophysiology was developed primarily for the second-year medical student. However, third- and fourth-year medical students, as well as house officers, may find this book to be useful, particularly when reviewing for board exams. Case histories and problems are integrated within the text. The reader should attempt to answer these questions before proceeding. We have assumed that the reader has a basic understanding of renal anatomy and histology. Although a previous introduction to renal physiology is helpful, it is not essential.

I am grateful to the many medical students at the University of Michigan who reviewed these chapters and provided many helpful comments.

James A. Shayman, MD

CONTENTS

Lippincott's Pathophysiology Series: Renal Pathophysiology, edited by James A. Shayman. J. B. Lippincott Company, Philadelphia © 1995.

Water

James A. Shayman

OBJECTIVES

By the end of this chapter the reader should be able to:

- Distinguish between osmolality and tonicity.
- Calculate plasma osmolality from plasma sodium, glucose, and blood urea nitrogen (BUN) concentrations. Understand the difference between calculated and measured plasma osmolality.
- Understand the basic physiology of osmoregulation and vasopressin release.
- Define and calculate free-water clearance.
- Distinguish between the separate actions of vasopressin on tubular water transport and vasoconstriction.
- Understand the role of tubular countercurrent transport in establishing renal osmolar gradients and its importance in antidiuresis.
- List the major causes of pseudohyponatremia.
- List causes of hyponatremia associated with appropriately low urine osmolalities.
- List causes of hyponatremia associated with high urine osmolalities. Distinguish between causes associated with decreased effective intra-arterial volume and causes associated with euvolemia.
- Calculate the water excess of a hyponatremic patient.
- Distinguish between central and nephrogenic diabetes insipidus.
- Calculate the water deficit of a hypernatremic patient.

The regulation of the *composition* of an organism's intracellular and extracellular fluid compartments is critical for life. Water balance is central to the determination of fluid compartment composition. Unlike the measurement of other biologically important compounds such as calcium, sodium, or glucose, the measurement of water concentration is made indirectly. Changes in water concentration are detected as changes in solute concentration (i.e., plasma osmolality). The higher the plasma osmolality, the lower the concentration of water in the plasma. Conversely, the lower the plasma osmolality, the higher the concentration of water in the plasma. The major contributent to plasma osmolality is sodium; therefore, patients who suffer from derangements in water metabolism typically present with either hyponatremia or hypernatremia. Understanding the pathophysiology of disorders of sodium concentration is, for all practical purposes, equivalent to understanding the pathophysiology of water metabolism and osmoregulation. The physiologic basis for osmoregulation and the approach to the patient with disorders of water metabolism (i.e., hyponatremia or hypernatremia) is the focus of this chapter.

PHYSIOLOGY OF OSMOREGULATION

MEASUREMENTS OF SOLUTE AND WATER CONCENTRATION

A compartment is separated by a membrane that is permeable to water but not solute (Fig. 1-1). If one side contains water only, and the other side contains water and solute, then water will move from an area of high concentration (i.e., the side without solute) to an area of lower concentration (i.e., the side with solute). The hydrostatic pressure (π) that the movement of water exerts is termed the osmotic pressure. The osmotic pressure is defined by van't Hoff's law: $\pi = nCRT$, where n represents the number of dissociable particles per molecule, C equals the solute concentration, R equals the gas constant and T equals tempera-

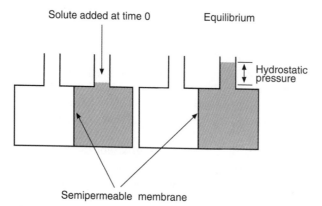

Figure 1-1. Hydrostatic pressure is generated as a result of an osmotic gradient. Solute applied to the right side of the tank results in the movement of water across a semipermeable membrane. The hydrostatic pressure measured by the change in column height is proportionate to the osmotic pressure of the solution.

ture in degrees kelvin. Osmotic pressure is independent of the actual properties of the solute particles, such as size or valence.

Expressing osmotic pressure measurements in units of atmosphere or mm Hg is not particularly useful for managing patients. For clinical purposes, osmotic pressure is redefined in units of osmolarity, or the concentration of solute particles per unit volume. Because water will move across most cellular membranes from a compartment of high concentration to a compartment of lower concentration, the solute concentration or osmolarity is an indirect measure of water concentration. In other words, *the higher the osmolarity, the lower the water concentration.*

The identical concentration of different solutes may contribute unequally to osmolarity, because some solutes will dissociate in solution, whereas other solutes will not. Two of the major solutes in plasma are sodium chloride and glucose. The osmotic pressure exerted by equal concentrations of each of these solutes will be quite different. Sodium chloride dissociates almost completely, whereas glucose does not. The osmotic pressure exerted by glucose will be only one half of that exerted by sodium chloride. Thus, a 300 mmolar solution of glucose will have an osmolarity of 300 mOsm/L, but a 300 mmolar solution of sodium chloride will have an osmolarity of 600 mOsm/L. Because the volume of water varies with temperature, and because the volume of plasma is comprised of only approximately 94% water, the concentration of osmoles is commonly expressed in terms of the weight of water. This value is termed the *osmolality* and is expressed in units of mOsm/kg water.

Cellular membranes vary in their permeability properties to different solutes. A solution of high osmolarity may greatly affect the movement of water across a cellular membrane if the membrane is impermeant to the solute. Conversely, a solution of equally high osmolarity may have little or no effect on water movement if the membrane is freely permeable to the solute present. The property of a solution that describes its ability to cause water movement into or out of a cell is referred to as *tonicity.* Exposing tissues to hypertonic solutions will cause them to shrink; exposing tissues to hypotonic solutions will result in swelling. The contribution of a given solute to the tonicity of a solution will therefore depend on its permeability characteristics.

Several solutes are routinely measured in plasma (Table 1-1). Sodium is present in high concentration. Although many cells have sodium channels and transporters that allow for the movement of sodium down a concentration gradient, the Na^+, K^+-ATPase transporter present on all cells actively extrudes sodium from inside cells and actively transports potassium from outside cells. Thus, cells are thought of as being relatively impermeant to sodium. Sodium is a large contributor to both plasma osmolarity and tonicity and is termed an *effective osmole.* Another solute that is present in plasma in relatively high concentrations is urea. Urea is freely permeable across most cell membranes as a result of the presence of a transporter that facilitates its movement down a concentration gradient. High levels of plasma urea seen in patients with chronic renal failure contribute little to the movement of water from intracellular to extracellular compartments. Urea therefore contributes to plasma osmolarity but contributes little to plasma tonicity. Urea is considered to be an *ineffective osmole.*

In practical terms, the only fluid compartment that is readily accessible for measurements of osmolarity is the intravascular compartment. The plasma osmolarity is easily and routinely measured in clinical laboratories. By knowing which extracellular solutes contribute most significantly to the plasma osmotic pressure,

TABLE 1-1. *SERUM SOLUTE CONCENTRATIONS*				
SUBSTANCE	**MOLECULAR WEIGHT**	**EQ/MOLE**	**OSM/MOLE**	**PLASMA CONCENTRATION**
Na^+	23	1	1	135–145 mEq/L
K^+	39.1	1	1	3.5–4.5 mEq/L
Cl^-	35.5	1	1	95–105 mEq/L
HCO_3^-	61	1	1	24–32 mEq/L
Ca^{++}	40.1	2	1	9.0–10.3 mg/dl (2.25–2.57 mmol/L)
PO_4^{-3}	95	3	1	3.5–4.5 mg/dl (1.12–1.45 mmole/L)
NH_4^+	18	1	1	10.6–28.2 µmol/L
Glucose	180		1	65–110 mg/dl (3.57–6.05 mmol/L)
Urea	60		1	8–25 mg/dl

the plasma osmolality can be calculated to closely approximate the clinically measured value. The normal concentrations for major plasma solutes are listed in Table 1-1. Ions such as sodium, potassium, chloride, and bicarbonate are usually expressed as mEq/L to more accurately reflect the stoichiometry of the interaction between cations and anions. For ions such as calcium or phosphate, which have more than one equivalent per mole, the concentration expressed in terms of osmolality will be proportionately lower. Solutes such as glucose and urea are conventionally expressed in mg/dl. To convert the concentrations of these solutes to mOsm/L, a conversion factor must be employed. The plasma osmolality may be calculated by using the following equation:

$$P_{Osm} = 2 \times [Na^+]_p + [glucose\ (mg/dl)]/18 + [BUN\ (mg/dl)]/2.8 \qquad [1-1]$$

The sodium concentration is multiplied by 2 because the cationic charge must be balanced by an equal concentration of anions (primarily chloride and bicarbonate).

PROBLEM 1

Calculate the normal plasma osmolality based on the values provided in Table 1-1. Calculate the relative contribution of sodium and its associated anions to overall plasma osmolality.

ANSWER: The calculated osmolality is 290 mOsm/kg water. Sodium and its associated anions (primarily chloride and bicarbonate) represent 96.5% of the calculated osmolality.

The difference between the measured and calculated osmolality represents potassium and other unmeasured osmoles. These osmoles, under normal conditions, contribute no more than 10 mOsm/kg water to the measured osmolality. The difference between measured and calculated osmolality is referred to as the *osmolar gap*.

The plasma sodium concentration is the major determinant of the plasma osmolality. Patients with measured plasma sodium concentrations of less than 135 mEq/L should be considered to have hypoosmolar disorders; those with plasma sodium concentrations of greater than 145 mEq/L should be considered to have hyperosmolar disorders. Stated differently, *a low plasma sodium concentration reflects a high plasma water concentration; a high plasma sodium concentration reflects a low plasma water concentration.*

REGULATION OF OSMOLALITY

Several types of detector and effector mechanisms exist for the preservation of sodium homeostasis (see Chap. 2). In contrast, the regulation of body fluid osmolality or water metabolism is accomplished by a single detector, the *hypothalamic osmoreceptor*, and by only two effector pathways, *thirst* and *renal water clearance*. Water clearance is regulated by *antidiuretic hormone* (ADH).

Changes in body fluid osmolality are detected by osmoreceptors located in the supraoptic and paraventricular nuclei of the hypothalamus. These osmoreceptors respond to changes in the concentration of effective osmoles by stimulating one of two responses. One set of osmoreceptors stimulates neural receptors involved in thirst. The second set of osmoreceptors stimulates the release of ADH from the posterior lobe of the pituitary gland. Hypertonicity is a very potent stimulus to the activation of both thirst and ADH release. Changes in plasma osmolality by as little as 2% above normal are sufficient to stimulate both effector responses. Changes in intravascular volume are also capable of stimulating both thirst and ADH release. However, a change in blood volume of at least 10% is usually required to elicit an increase in plasma antidiuretic hormone levels. ADH release is regulated by factors other than osmolality and volume. These factors are listed in Table 1-2.

Volume (or blood pressure) and osmolality-induced changes in ADH release may be interactive. Figure 1-2 shows the relation among plasma ADH levels (y axis), plasma osmolality (x axis), and volume (or blood pressure). Changes in volume or pressure affect ADH levels in two ways. These changes alter the slope of the line that relates ADH levels to osmolality. In other words, the patient who is hy-

TABLE 1-2. *EFFECTORS OF ANTIDIURETIC HORMONE SECRETION*

STIMULATORY	INHIBITORY
Hyperosmolality	Hypoosmolality
Hypovolemia or hypotension	Hypervolemia or hypertension
Nausea	Atrial natriuretic hormone
Angiotensin II	
Drugs (e.g., nicotine, narcotics, vincristine, cyclophosphamide, chlorpropamide)	Drugs (e.g., ethanol, narcotic antagonists, phenytoin)

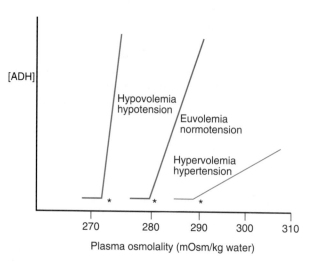

Figure 1-2. Association between plasma antidiuretic hormone (ADH) concentration, osmotic-dependent stimuli, and volume-dependent stimuli. (*, set point for ADH secretion.)

potensive or hypovolemic will secrete a greater amount of ADH for a given increase in plasma osmolality compared with the patient who is normotensive and euvolemic. Changes in volume or blood pressure change the set point for ADH release. The *set point* is defined as the plasma osmolality at which plasma ADH levels begin to increase over baseline. Under normal circumstances, the set point for adults varies between 280 and 290 mOsm/kg water. The set point for ADH release may change under other conditions. Pregnancy, malnutrition, cancer, and psychosis are conditions associated with a lower set point for ADH release. The evaluation of patients with altered set points for ADH release is discussed later in the chapter.

ROLE OF THE KIDNEY IN REGULATING WATER METABOLISM

ADH is released from the posterior pituitary gland, circulates throughout the bloodstream, and exerts two physiologic effects. ADH induces vasoconstriction resulting in increased systemic vascular resistance. ADH binds to the distal tubule and stimulates the retention of water. The net result of the latter action is the formation of a concentrated urine of high osmolality, hence the name antidiuretic hormone. Thus, the greater the circulating level of ADH, the more concentrated the urine formed; the lower the level of ADH, the more dilute the urine formed. A high ADH level will increase urine osmolality and decrease water excretion but have no effect on solute excretion. This relation is displayed in Figure 1-3.

The ability of the kidney to separate solute and water excretion can be quantitated without knowledge of any of the specific mechanisms of urine water excretion. This can be accomplished by comparing the clearance of solute, the *osmolar clearance*, and of water, the *free-water clearance*.

Any compound (X) that is filtered by the kidney will be excreted into the urine at a given rate. The rate of excretion is proportional to the plasma concentration of X (P^a_X). The urinary excretion rate may be expressed as the product of the urinary concentration of X (U_X) and the urinary flow rate in ml/minute (V):

$$P^a_x \propto U_x \times V \qquad\qquad [1\text{-}2]$$

The factor that equates the urinary excretion of X with the arterial plasma concentration of X is the removal rate or *clearance* of X (C_x). The removal rate or clearance may be added to the equation:

$$P^a_x \times C_x = U_x \times V$$

Rearranged, the equation can be stated as follows:

$$C_x = (U_x \times V)/P^a_x$$

PROBLEM 2

Plasma creatinine concentration is 1 mg/dl. Urine creatinine concentration is 60 mg/dl. The 24-hour urine volume is 2880 ml. Calculate the clearance of creatinine.

ANSWER: The urine flow rate is (2880 ml/24 hours) × (24 hours/1440 minutes) = 2 ml/minute.

The urine creatinine concentration is
(60 mg/dl) × (1 dl/100 ml) = 0.6 mg/ml.

The plasma creatinine concentration is
(1 mg/dl) × (1 dl/100 ml) = 0.01 mg/ml.

The clearance of creatinine
$$\begin{aligned}(C_{creatinine}) &= (U_{creatinine} \times V)/(P_{creatinine}) \\ &= (2 \text{ ml/minute} \times 0.6 \text{ mg/ml})/(0.01 \text{ mg/ml}) \\ &= 120 \text{ ml/min}.\end{aligned}$$

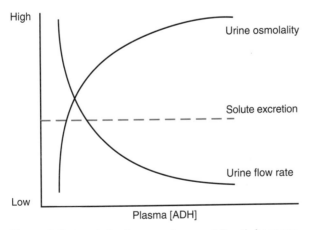

Figure 1-3. Association between plasma antidiuretic hormone (ADH) concentration, solute excretion, urine osmolality, and urine volume.

The values for the clearance of a given substance are expressed in units of volume per unit time. Conceptually, clearance represents the plasma volume from which this given substance has been removed by both filtration and secretion into the urine per unit time. Clearance depends on both the filtration rate of the substance in question and on the subsequent handling of the substance in the renal tubule. Since a given substance X may be either secreted or reabsorbed in the tubule, the concentration of X in the urine is a reflection of the net excretion and handling of X by the nephron.

Substituting the total solute concentration (i.e., osmolality) or water concentration for X permits the determination of the ability of the kidney to separate solute and water under conditions of water balance, water conservation, or water excretion.

PROBLEM 3

The following values are obtained for three different patients:

	Patient 1	**Patient 2**	**Patient 3**
P_{Osm}	300 mOsm/kg water	300 mOsm/kg water	300 mOsm/kg water
U_{Osm}	300 mOsm/kg water	150 mOsm/kg water	600 mOsm/kg water
Urine flow (ml/minute)	2 ml/minute	4 ml/minute	1 ml/minute

Patient 1 is in water balance; patient 2 is overhydrated; and patient 3 is dehydrated. For each patient, calculate the osmolar clearance (C_{Osm}).

ANSWER

$$C_{Osm} = (U_{Osm} \times V)/(P_{Osm})$$

Patient 1 $C_{Osm} = (300 \text{ mOsm/kg water} \times 2 \text{ ml/minute})/(300 \text{ mOsm/kg water}) = 2 \text{ ml/minute}$

Patient 2 $C_{Osm} = (150 \text{ mOsm/kg water} \times 4 \text{ ml/minute})/(300 \text{ mOsm/kg water}) = 2 \text{ ml/minute}$

Patient 3 $C_{Osm} = (600 \text{ mOsm/kg water} \times 1 \text{ ml/minute})/(300 \text{ mOsm/kg water}) = 2 \text{ ml/minute}$

In each patient, the clearance of solute is identical despite the existence of widely differing urine flow rates. In the first patient, who is in water balance, the osmolar clearance equals the urine flow rate. In the second patient, who is overhydrated, the urine flow rate exceeds the osmolar clearance. The difference between the urine flow rate and osmolar clearance represents the volume of solute-free water that has been excreted. Thus, the second patient is excreting solute-free water at a rate of 2 ml/minute ($V - C_{Osm}$ or 4 ml/minute − 2 ml/minute). This value, $V - C_{Osm}$, is referred to as the *free-water clearance*.

In the third patient, who is dehydrated, the difference between V and C_{Osm} (1 ml/minute − 2 ml/minute) is a negative number. This value represents solute-free water that has been reabsorbed by the kidneys and returned to the circulation. Stated differently, this value represents the volume of water per unit time which would have to be added to the urine to created a urine osmolality equal to that of the plasma. A negative free-water clearance is termed the *tubular conservation of water* (T^c_{water}).

For each patient, the clearance of solute is equal, therefore water clearance occurs independent of solute. In other words, there is net separation in the handling of solute and water by the kidney. The ability of the kidney to dissociate water and solute excretion is dependent on ADH.

CELLULAR EFFECTS OF ANTIDIURETIC HORMONE

ADH circulates throughout the bloodstream following its release from the posterior pituitary gland. This cyclic octapeptide has two primary sites of action (Fig. 1-4): the vascular smooth muscle cell and the kidney at the collecting duct. Binding of ADH to vascular smooth muscle is mediated by type 1 (V_1) vasopressin receptors and results in vascular smooth muscle contraction. Cell signaling occurs through the activation of phospholipase C, with the generation of inositol trisphosphate and diacylglycerol. Inositol trisphosphate results in the mobilization of intracellular calcium; diacylglycerol activates protein kinase C. These actions initiate a cascade of secondary signals that results in cellular contraction. Binding of ADH to the renal tubule is mediated by type 2 (V_2) vasopressin receptors. Renal ADH binding results in the activation of adenylyl cyclase, with the generation of cAMP and

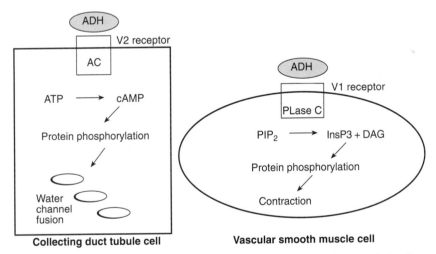

Figure 1-4. Cell signaling by antidiuretic hormone (ADH) in collecting duct tubule cells and vascular smooth muscle cells. In tubule cells, ADH binds to the V2 receptor on the basolateral membrane, generates cAMP from adenylyl cyclase (AC), and initiates a signaling cascade resulting in the insertion of water channels in the apical membrane. In smooth muscle cells, ADH binds to the V1 receptor, generates inositol trisphosphate (InsP3) and diacylglycerol (DAG), and initiates a signaling cascade resulting in cellular contraction. (ATP, adenosine triphosphate, PIP_2 phosphatidylinositol 4,5-bisphosphate.)

activation of protein kinase A. This signaling cascade results in the fusion of water channels with the plasma membrane, allowing for the movement of water from the tubular lumen to the bloodstream. The renal effects of ADH are critical for the ability of the kidney to concentrate the urine.

COUNTERCURRENT MULTIPLICATION AND WATER TRANSPORT

To understand how ADH acts as an effector for the maintenance of fluid osmolality, one must understand how the kidney, and more specifically the nephron, is able to generate either a concentrated (i.e., hyperosmotic) or dilute (i.e., hypoosmotic) urine. A limited number of general principles govern the contribution of the nephron to water clearance.

Water can move across membranes only passively. The formation of a urine of low osmolality requires the removal of solute to the exclusion of water in the nephron. Conversely, the formation of a urine of high osmolality requires the existence of a compartment where the solute concentration is greater than that of the plasma, allowing for water to move down its concentration gradient. The inner medullary area of the kidney serves this role. In this region of the kidney, the interstitial osmolality is capable of attaining concentrations of up to 1200 mOsm/kg water (Table 1-3). Under normal conditions, solute and water transport proceed in an ADH-independent manner.

The maximal level of dilution of the urine depends on the ability of the kidney to lower the osmolality of the tubular fluid. The lowering of tubular fluid osmolality is accomplished by highly active sodium chloride transport in the ascending limb and distal tubule. In the thick ascending limb, sodium chloride transport occurs by the $Na^+,K^+,2Cl^-$ cotransporter. In the distal tubule, a sodium chloride cotransporter is responsible for sodium chloride transport. In both segments, the energy driving sodium chloride transport is provided by the Na^+, K^+-ATPase located on the basolateral surface of the tubular cells. The $Na^+,K^+,2Cl^-$ cotransporter is sensitive to loop diuretics such as furosemide. The Na^+, Cl^- cotransporter is sensitive to thiazide diuretics. Thus, diuretic therapy will impair the ability of the kidney to generate a maximally dilute urine.

If the tubular fluid osmolality at the beginning of the collecting duct is 100

TABLE 1-3. *TUBULAR FLUID OSMOLALITY (mOsm/kg WATER) AT NEPHRON SITES UNDER CONDITIONS OF MINIMAL OR MAXIMAL ANTIDIURETIC HORMONE (ADH) EFFECT*

NEPHRON SEGMENT	NO ADH	MAXIMAL ADH
Proximal tubule	300	300
Start of descending thin limb	300	300
Start of ascending thin limb	1200	1200
End of thick ascending limb	100	100
End of cortical collecting duct	50–100	300
Final urine	50	1200

mOsm/kg water and no ADH is present, urine osmolality will be maintained at 100 mOsm/kg water or less as a result of additional sodium chloride transport in the collecting duct. In the presence of ADH, water channels in the collecting tubule are inserted into the plasma membrane, allowing water to move into the medullary interstium. Under conditions of maximal ADH activity, the tubular fluid is able to attain an osmolality equivalent to the interstitium, resulting in antidiuresis and the excretion of a hyperosmolar urine.

The formation of a concentrated urine depends on the presence of a high medullary interstitial osmolality. Understanding how water can leave the tubule to form a concentrated urine requires insight into the mechanism of solute concentration in the renal medulla. Such insight can be gained by comparing the renal anatomy of various animal species with their ability to generate concentrated urines. Diagrammatic representations of nephrons from amphibians, birds, and mammals are displayed in Figure 1-5. Nephrons from birds and mammals contain loop structures, whereas nephrons from amphibians and almost all other species do not. Amphibians, reptiles, birds, and mammals are all comparable in their ability to generate low urine osmolalities compared to plasma osmolalities. However, only birds and mammals are able to generate urine osmolalities that are high relative to their plasma osmolalities. Because the degree of ionic transport or ionic gradient that an individual cell can generate is comparable between nephron segments of different species, the capacity to form a concentrated urine must depend on the unique anatomic characteristics of bird and mammalian nephrons. The role of the loop of Henle in forming a concentrated urine can be explained by the process of *countercurrent multiplication.*

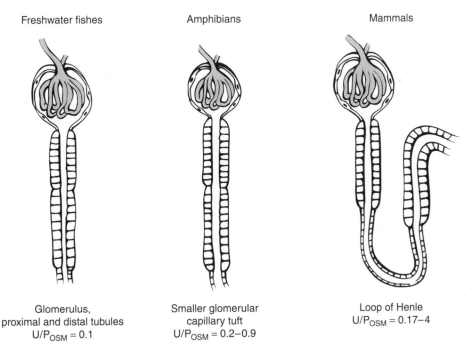

Freshwater fishes Amphibians Mammals

Glomerulus, proximal and distal tubules
$U/P_{OSM} = 0.1$

Smaller glomerular capillary tuft
$U/P_{OSM} = 0.2–0.9$

Loop of Henle
$U/P_{OSM} = 0.17–4$

Figure 1-5. Comparative anatomy of the nephron. U/P_{Osm} denotes the ratio of urine osmolality to plasma osmolality.

Contribution of the Loop of Henle

The descending limb of the loop of Henle has very high water permeability and relatively low active sodium chloride transport and passive sodium chloride permeability. The ascending limb is effectively impermeant to water but possesses a relatively high sodium chloride transport capacity. The result of these segment-specific differences in transport characteristics is shown in Figure 1-6. If at some theoretical time 0 there is no medullary osmotic gradient, then fluid entering the descending limb will have an osmolality equal to that of plasma filtrate. There is no tubular-to-interstitial osmotic concentration gradient; therefore, no net movement of water from the descending limb to the interstitium occurs. As the tubular fluid enters the ascending limb, however, sodium transport creates an interstitial-to-ascending tubule osmotic gradient proportionate to the degree of sodium chloride transport. Tubular fluid entering the descending limb will have an osmolality that is lower than that of the interstium. Water will passively move from an area of high concentration or low osmolality (i.e., the descending limb) to an area of low concentration or high osmolality (i.e., the interstitium). Sodium chloride transport continues in the ascending limb, however, and the medullary osmotic concentration continues to rise. If this process is repeated several times, the interstitial osmolality will rise significantly, to 1200 mOsm/kg water versus 300 mOsm/kg water in

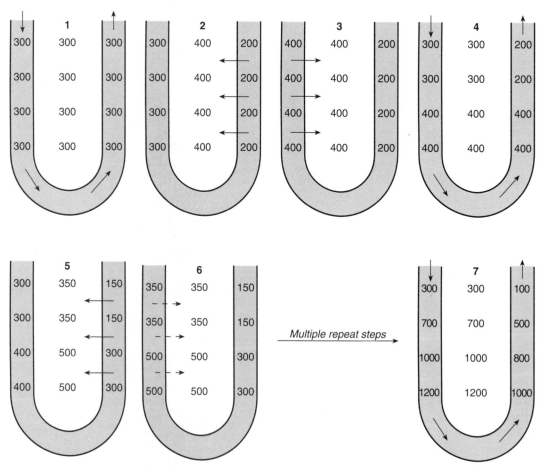

Figure 1-6. Countercurrent multiplication.

plasma. Thus, the cortical-to-medullary osmotic gradient created by countercurrent multiplication (~900 mOsm/kg water) is impressively large; the gradient contributed by the ascending limb (~200 mOsm/kg water) to generate this high interstitial osmolality is modest.

Sodium and chloride are not the only contributors to the interstitial osmolality. Urea contributes approximately one half of the interstitial osmolality. Urea accumulation in the medullary interstitium occurs as a result of two primary factors. Urea is transported across the tubular epithelium by passive permeability, and transport occurs in the presence of a concentration gradient. There is no active transport of urea. The thick ascending limb, distal convoluted tubule, and cortical collecting duct are impermeant to urea. The medullary collecting duct has a very high urea permeability. The thin descending and ascending limb tubular segments are also urea permeable, albeit to a lesser degree than the medullary collecting tubule. Tubular urea concentration rises as filtrate moves from the loop of Henle through the distal convoluted and cortical collecting tubules as a result of the movement of water to the exclusion of urea in these segments. As fluid enters the inner medullary tubule, an area where passive permeability is high, urea moves from the tubule to the medullary interstitium. However, because the medullary interstitial urea concentration is greater than the tubular concentration in Henle's loop, urea is transported from the interstitium back to the tubule. The consequence of this selective permeability of the tubule to urea is the cycling of urea from the tubule to the interstitium.

DISORDERS OF PLASMA OSMOLALITY: THE HYPONATREMIC PATIENT

Plasma consists primarily of water. Other components include low-molecular-weight solutes (e.g., sodium, potassium, chloride, bicarbonate, urea, glucose) and higher-molecular-weight compounds (e.g., plasma proteins, lipids). Electrolytes carry a charge, and therefore they distribute almost exclusively into water. High-molecular-weight compounds are nonpolar by comparison. These proteins and lipids constitute a significant fraction of the total volume of plasma (~6%–7%); therefore, these compounds exclude electrolytes from the volume of plasma which they occupy.

PROBLEM 4

Calculate the plasma concentration of sodium in a patient with a measured sodium of 143 mEq/L based exclusively on the distribution of sodium into the polar, aqueous component of plasma.

ANSWER: When the plasma concentration of a particular solute such as Na or Cl is measured, the clinical laboratory expresses the concentration per volume of plasma. However, the concentration of sodium *per liter of water* is greater. One liter of plasma consists of 930 ml of water; therefore, the sodium concentration equals 143/0.93 = 154 mEq/L *water*. This in fact is the concentration of sodium in 0.9% saline (otherwise referred to as normal saline). The physiologic replacement of sodium chloride is based on the distribution of sodium into the aqueous compartment of plasma.

Some patients suffer from abnormalities of lipid or protein metabolism that lower the fraction of plasma comprised of water. Hypertriglyceridemia and hypercholesterolemia, if sufficiently severe, decrease the fraction of plasma comprised of water, and plasma sodium concentration is reported as abnormally low. However, the plasma sodium concentration expressed as mEq/L *water* is normal. Similarly, the plasma osmolality expressed as mOsm/kg *water* is normal. The hypothalamic osmoreceptors detect a normal solute concentration in the plasma. Some plasma proteins are very hydrophobic and exclude water. Waldenström's macroglobulinemia is a lymphoproliferative disorder associated with increased production of IgM-type immunoglobulin. Patients with high plasma IgM levels may also have apparently low plasma sodium concentrations.

Patients that have falsely low measured plasma sodium concentrations are said to have *pseudohyponatremia.* Hyperlipidemia and hyperproteinemia are two causes of pseudohyponatremia. Because hyponatremia can be operationally equated with hypoosmolality, pseudohyponatremia can be more broadly defined. *A patient with pseudohyponatremia has a low measured plasma sodium concentration in the setting of a normal or high plasma osmolality.*

This principle is illustrated in Case 1.

CASE 1

A 70-year-old woman with a five-year history of non–insulin-dependent diabetes mellitus arrives at the emergency department with mental status changes. On physical examination, her blood pressure is 120/80 mm Hg, her pulse is 70 bpm and regular, and her respiratory rate is 18 breaths per minute. Her skin turgor is normal, and there are no signs of dehydration. Her cardiovascular and respiratory examinations are normal. The neurologic examination reveals the absence of any focal findings. The serum electrolytes are as follows:

Sodium	125 mEq/L
Chloride	90 mEq/L
Potassium	4.0 mEq/L
Bicarbonate	22 mEq/L
Glucose	720 mg/dl
BUN	14 mg/dl

CASE DISCUSSION

In trying to determine why this patient is hyponatremic, the plasma osmolality can be calculated based on the measured solute. Previously, the calculated osmolality was defined as:

$$P_{Osm} = 2 \times [Na^+]_p + [glucose\ (mg/dl)]/18 + [BUN\ (mg/dl)]/2.8 \qquad [1\text{-}3]$$

Substituting the laboratory values from this patient:

$$P_{Osm} = 2 \times 125 + 720/18 + 14/2.8 = 250 + 40 + 5$$
$$= 295\ mOsm/L$$

This patient has a normal or slightly high osmolality. The hyponatremia is present because her hypothalamic osmoreceptors detect a high plasma solute concentration and therefore continue to signal the pituitary gland to release ADH. Because hyponatremia is equated with hypoosmolality in this text, hyperglycemia can be considered to be another cause of pseudohyponatremia. Many physicians restrict the use of the term pseudohyponatremia to cases of hyperlipidemia or hyperproteinemia. Because plasma sodium concentration normally reflects plasma osmolality, the broader definition used in this text is instructionally useful.

A second example of hyponatremia in the setting of normal osmolality is illustrated in Case 2.

CASE 2

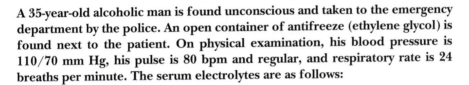

A 35-year-old alcoholic man is found unconscious and taken to the emergency department by the police. An open container of antifreeze (ethylene glycol) is found next to the patient. On physical examination, his blood pressure is 110/70 mm Hg, his pulse is 80 bpm and regular, and respiratory rate is 24 breaths per minute. The serum electrolytes are as follows:

Sodium	120 mEq/L
Potassium	4.0 mEq/L
Chloride	80 mEq/L
Bicarbonate	15 mEq/L
Glucose	90 mg/dl
BUN	14 mg/dl

CASE DISCUSSION

The calculated plasma osmolality for this patient is:

$$P_{Osm} = 2 \times 120 + 90/18 + 14/2.8 = 240 + 5 + 5$$
$$= 250 \text{ mOsm/L}$$

[1-4]

This value is clearly abnormally low. However, when a blood sample is sent to the laboratory for the direct measurement of plasma osmolality, a value of 290 mOsm/kg water is obtained. Previously it was determined that the difference between the measured osmolality and the calculated osmolality, the *osmolar gap*, normally did not exceed 10 mOsm/kg water. In this patient, the osmolar gap is 40 mOsm/kg water. The extra solute in the patient's plasma is the result of the ethylene glycol in the antifreeze. This solute contributes to the osmolality detected at the hypothalamus in the same manner that the abnormally high glucose did in the first case. However, ethylene glycol represents an unmeasured osmole. The presence of unmeasured osmoles is detected by comparing the measured plasma osmolality to the calculated plasma osmolality. Determining what the unmeasured osmoles actually are requires a good patient history and laboratory documentation with tests that assay the particular osmole. The low bicarbonate concentration is the result of the metabolism of ethylene glycol to glycolic and glyoxylic acids.

Cases of pseudohyponatremia represent conditions in which the plasma osmolality is normal or high and the patient's ability to sense changes in osmolality and respond to the detected plasma osmolality by altering the thirst response or renal water clearance is intact. Disorders of true hyponatremia, in contrast, represent conditions in which a derangement exists in the osmostat, thirst response, ADH release, or renal response to ADH. Diagnosing the basis for true hyponatremia can be challenging but is much less difficult when approached systematically. After pseudohyponatremia has been ruled out as a possible reason for hyponatremia, it is helpful to ask, "Is the renal response to hyponatremia (i.e., hypoosmolality) appropriate?"

If the plasma water concentration is too high, the kidney should respond by increasing the clearance of free water. As discussed previously, circulating ADH levels are suppressed, a dilute urine enters the collecting tubule, and water is unable to move from the collecting tubule to the renal medullary interstitium. This sequence of events is detected as a dilute urine. The simplest method for measuring urinary dilution is its specific gravity. A more accurate means of measuring urine water content is the measurement of urine osmolality. The urine osmolality at which there is neither free-water clearance nor tubular conservation of water is approximately 300 mOsm/kg water, the same as normal plasma osmolality. The corresponding urine specific gravity would be about 1.008.

A patient is mildly hyponatremic; his plasma sodium is 128 mEq/L. If the patient's urine osmolality is measured and it is discovered that it is appropriately low (for example, 150 mOsm/kg water), then it can be concluded that the patient's kidneys are capable of generating a dilute urine. ADH levels are also suppressed. The cause of the hyponatremia and hypoosmolality probably involves some aspect of water metabolism other than the kidney or the formation or release of ADH. Because of the simplicity of the axis which controls water metabolism, we can conclude that the derangement must exist in either osmoreceptor function or the thirst response.

A classic example of an individual with normal osmoreceptor function, ADH release, and renal response to ADH is the patient with *psychogenic polydipsia*. These patients exhibit a compulsion to drink excessively large amounts of water. The occurrence of hyponatremia in the setting of polydipsia is rare, because normally, an adult can drink 20 L of water per day without the development of fluid retention or hyponatremia. More often, these patients become hyponatremic when they have some coexisting limitation of water excretion, such as the use of diuretics.

Another example of a patient with a normal ability of the kidney to excrete free water is illustrated in Case 3.

CASE 3

A 25-year-old woman presents to her obstetrician in her twelfth week of pregnancy. Her pregravid plasma Na was 144 mEq/L, and plasma osmolality was 290 mOsm/kg water. Repeat plasma sodium is 132 mEq/L, and plasma osmolality is 278 mOsm/kg water.

CASE DISCUSSION

Pregnancy is commonly associated with mild hyponatremia and hypoosmolality. Hyponatremia begins at about the fifth week postconception and reaches its nadir by the tenth week of pregnancy. This is the result of a lowering of the osmotic threshold for vasopressin release and thirst suppression. This phenomenon is referred to as a *reset osmostat*. Other clinical conditions associated with hyponatremia as a result of a reset osmostat include malnutrition and psychosis.

Vasopressin release is not only regulated by plasma osmolality but is also affected by the *effective circulating blood volume*. The effective circulating volume is the part of the extracellular fluid that is effectively perfusing tissues and stimulating volume receptors. Under normal circumstances, the circulating blood volume is directly proportionate to the extracellular volume. Thus, a patient who is sodium loaded will expand his or her extracellular volume and increase his or her effective circulating blood volume. Conversely, the sodium depleted patient will decrease his or her extracellular volume and similarly decrease his or her circulating blood volume. In the case of sodium depletion, a volume- or pressure-dependent stimulation of vasopressin release occurs. Examples of such cases include the patient who is hypotensive as a result of blood loss, and the patient who is severely dehydrated as a result of excessive diarrhea or sweating. This is a protective response. The elevated vasopressin stimulates the transport of water in the distal tubule, resulting in the prevention of additional losses of extracellular volume. Vasopressin also stimulates vasoconstriction and thus maintains blood pressure.

Often, however, extracellular fluid volume is not proportionate to the effective circulating volume. Case 4 illustrates such an example.

CASE 4

A 50-year-old man visits his internist with complaints of weight gain and edema of his lower limbs. He notes that his waist has expanded to the point where his belts no longer fit. He admits to drinking a fifth of whiskey each day. His normal weight is 70 kg; he now weighs 110 kg. On physical examination, his blood pressure is 110/70 mm Hg without orthostatic changes. His skin reveals spider angiomata and palmar erythema. His neck reveals no jugular venous distention. His chest is clear to auscultation and his cardiovascular exam is negative. On abdominal examination, he has marked distention with shifting dullness. The extremities show 4+ edema in his thighs. There is also testicular atrophy. Laboratory examination is significant for the following.

Sodium	125 mEq/L
Chloride	90 mEq/L
Total protein	5.3 g/dl
Potassium	4.0 mEq/L
Bicarbonate	22 mEq/L
Albumin	2 g/dl
Glucose	80 mg/dl
BUN	4 mg/dl

CASE DISCUSSION

This patient has alcohol-induced cirrhosis. His examination reveals massive hypervolemia with signs of ascites and lower-extremity edema due to portal hypertension. Such patients are commonly hyponatremic and have true hypoosmolality. Because cirrhotic patients lack normal hepatic synthetic function, plasma protein concentrations, specifically plasma albumin levels, are decreased. This results in a lower plasma oncotic pressure (see Chap. 2) and thus a lower effective circulating volume. These patients thus have stimuli for both water and sodium retention. ADH levels are elevated as a result of a change in the set point for ADH release and the volume-dependent stimulus, resulting in both vasoconstriction and renal water transport. The decrease in effective blood volume also results in a fall in glomerular filtration rate (GFR) and an elevation in renin levels. Renin will stimulate angiotensin II and aldosterone formation, resulting in distal tubular sodium transport.

Two other clinical syndromes are commonly associated with hyponatremia in the setting of hypervolemia. In congestive heart failure, a fall in cardiac output results in a decrease in effective tissue perfusion. In nephrotic syndrome (see Chap. 5), the nephrotic patient suffers from protein loss with similar abnormally low levels of plasma albumin and total protein. This is in contrast to the cirrhotic patient in whom the primary defect is in protein synthesis. In each syndrome, stimuli for ADH release, renin release and sodium retention exist as a result of a decreased GFR and increased aldosterone.

In the general case of either hypovolemia- or hypervolemia-associated hypoosmolality, two laboratory parameters are informative. The first is the urine osmolality. In both conditions, there is true hypoosmolality. The appropriate response by the kidney ought to be the clearance of free water from the body; thus, the urine osmolality should be low. However, because a decrease in the effective circulating volume serves as a stimulus for ADH release in both hypovolemia and hypervolemia, the measured urine osmolalities will be inappropriately high (e.g., >200 mOsm/kg water).

The second useful laboratory measurement is the urine sodium. Because a decrease in effective circulating volume serves as a stimulus for sodium retention, the measured urine sodium concentration will be low (e.g., <10 mEq/L). Both of these tests are useful in establishing that hyponatremia is the result of a decrease in effective circulating volume.

A common feature of each of the cases illustrated previously is that the ability of the kidney to respond normally to a water load is not impaired. The basis for the development of hyponatremia is the result of some other defect (e.g., an abnormal response of the osmoreceptors, impaired organ perfusion). In some cases of hyponatremia, however, there is an impairment in renal water excretion. The obvious case is that of chronic renal failure. If renal function is sufficiently impaired, the ability of the kidney to respond to a water load by excreting excess free water is limited. Impaired renal water excretion also is observed with the use of diuretics, typically thiazides. With diuretic use, the ability of the thick ascending limb of Henle and the distal tubule to reabsorb sodium and thereby generate a maximally dilute urine is limited. The degree of free-water excretion is dependent on the degree to which the urine osmolality can be lowered in these tubular segments.

In contrast with the examples of hyponatremia detailed previously, in which patients are typically hypovolemic or volume overloaded, other cases of hypoosmolality are associated with euvolemia. These cases are typified by the nonphysiologic secretion of ADH. Nonphysiologic refers to the fact that there is neither an osmotic stimulus (i.e., hyperosmolality) nor a volume stimulus (i.e., decreased effective circulating volume) for ADH release. Two defined settings in which hyponatremia occurs in the absence of osmotic and volume stimuli are hypothyroidism and glucocorticoid deficiency. In both cases, circulating levels of ADH are high.

Another setting in which hyponatremia occurs is illustrated in Case 5.

CASE 5

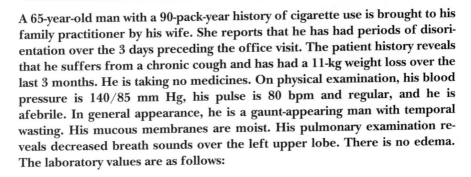

A 65-year-old man with a 90-pack-year history of cigarette use is brought to his family practitioner by his wife. She reports that he has had periods of disorientation over the 3 days preceding the office visit. The patient history reveals that he suffers from a chronic cough and has had a 11-kg weight loss over the last 3 months. He is taking no medicines. On physical examination, his blood pressure is 140/85 mm Hg, his pulse is 80 bpm and regular, and he is afebrile. In general appearance, he is a gaunt-appearing man with temporal wasting. His mucous membranes are moist. His pulmonary examination reveals decreased breath sounds over the left upper lobe. There is no edema. The laboratory values are as follows:

Sodium	115 mEq/L
Chloride	80 mEq/L
Glucose	80 mg/dl
Potassium	4.0 mEq/L
Bicarbonate	22 mEq/L
BUN	14 mg/dl
P_{Osm}	250 mOsm/kg water
U_{Osm}	80 mOsm/kg water

The patient's chest radiograph is significant for a 6-cm mass in the left upper lobe. Sputum cytology is subsequently obtained and is positive for small cell carcinoma.

CASE DISCUSSION

By comparing the calculated plasma osmolality to the measured plasma osmolality, it can be determined that the patient is truly hypoosmolar. The urine osmolality is inappropriately high for an individual who should be eliminating free water from his body. This patient is neither hypovolemic nor hypervolemic. This patient suffers from an excess of circulating ADH. He has the *syndrome of inappropriate secretion of ADH (SIADH)*. This syndrome has been identified in association with a wide spectrum of diseases. In general, however, the associated diseases fall into three general categories: malignancies, central nervous system disorders, and pulmonary infections. A limited compilation of diseases associated with SIADH is given in Table 1-4.

TABLE 1-4. *CAUSES OF THE SYNDROME OF INAPPROPRIATE ANTIDIURETIC HORMONE SECRETION*

Ectopic antidiuretic hormone	Lung cancer (e.g., oat cell carcinoma, bronchogenic carcinoma), pancreatic carcinoma, leukemia, Hodgkin's lymphoma, thymoma
Central nervous system disorders	Brain tumors, encephalitis, meningitis, head trauma, lupus cerebritis
Pulmonary diseases	Pneumonia (i.e., viral or bacterial), tuberculosis, abscess

Finally, hyponatremia in the setting of euvolemia can result from any of a variety of drugs. Many drugs increase ADH release and thus impair renal free-water excretion. These include tricyclic antidepressants, nicotine, morphine, and the chemotherapeutic agents vincristine and cyclophosphamide. Other agents enhance the action of ADH. These include nonsteroidal antiinflammatory agents (e.g., ibuprofen, indomethacin) and sulfonylureas.

Evaluating patients with hyponatremia is often difficult; however, by sequentially asking three questions in each case, the diagnostic possibilities can be limited considerably.

1. *Does the patient have true hypoosmolality?* This question is answered by comparing the calculated plasma osmolality to the measured plasma osmolality and by ruling out the presence of hyperlipidemia or hyperproteinemia.

2. *If the patient suffers from true hypoosmolality, then is the kidney responding by clearing excess free water?* A hyponatremic patient ought to have a low urine osmolality, reflecting an appropriate response by the kidney to clear free water.

3. *Is there renal conservation of sodium?* A patient with a decreased effective circulating volume, whether the result of conditions associated with hypervolemia (e.g., nephrotic syndrome) or hypovolemia (e.g., dehydration), will usually conserve sodium.

PROBLEM 5

Match the laboratory values with the patient history.

	Na^+	K^+	Cl^-	HCO_3^-	Glucose	BUN	P_{Osm}	U_{Osm}	U_{Na}
1	125	4.5	80	35	90	30	268	450	<10
2	128	4.0	88	28	85	14	295	250	30
3	125	5.5	90	18	90	74	295	280	40
4	120	4.2	90	20	88	14	260	200	20

A. *A woman with long-standing hypertension and chronic renal failure.*
B. *A severely dehydrated man suffering from chronic vomiting.*

(continued)

C. *An immunosuppresed patient with fungal pneumonia.*
D. *A cardiac catheterization patient who received 100 g of mannitol at the time of his dye infusion.*

ANSWERS

1. *B.* The measured osmolality reveals that the patient is truly hypoosmolar. The urine osmolarity is high and the urine sodium is low, consistent with the retention of both water and sodium by the kidneys.

2. *D.* The calculated plasma osmolality is 266 mOsm/kg water. The measured osmolality is 295 mOsm/kg water. There is a large osmolar gap. Mannitol is an unmeasured osmole, commonly given during radiologic dye studies to protect the kidneys from the toxic effects of the radiocontrast agents.

3. *A.* The elevated BUN is consistent with chronic renal insufficiency. The hyponatremia is the result of the patient's inability to excrete free water because of renal impairment. Because urea is an ineffective osmole, the measured plasma osmolarity overestimates the effective osmolarity of the patient's plasma.

4. *C.* The calculated plasma osmolality and the measured plasma osmolarity are both low, indicating that the patient suffers from true hyponatremia. The urine osmolarity is inappropriately high, allowing psychogenic polydipsia or reset osmostat to be ruled out as potential causes of the hyponatremia. The high urine sodium is inconsistent with a decrease in effective circulating volume as the stimulus for ADH release. This case is consistent with SIADH, hypothyroidism, or adrenal insufficiency. A fungal pneumonia could be a cause of SIADH and the basis for the hyponatremia.

The clinical symptoms of hyponatremia are primarily neurologic and develop as a result of the movement of water into the central nervous system. It is unusual for patients to be symptomatic with plasma sodium concentrations greater than 125 mEq/L. Below this value, a spectrum of symptoms may be manifested, ranging from confusion and stupor to coma and seizures. The severity of the neurologic symptoms is dependent not only on the degree of hyponatremia but also on the rapidity with which the hyponatremia develops. High mortality rates are associated with significant hyponatremia that develops in less than 24 hours.

The approach to treating a hyponatremic patient varies depending on the underlying etiology of the condition. Therefore, it is not only important to identify the presence of hyponatremia but also to understand its pathogenesis. The choice of therapy depends on the patient's condition and the goals of treatment. The underlying condition should be identified and treated (e.g., diabetes, adrenal insufficiency, drug therapy). With regard to the hyponatremia, treatment varies from simple observation to aggressive correction. In some cases, no therapy should be initiated. For example, if a patient with congestive heart failure is compensated and the hyponatremia is mild, the physician may elect to simply observe the patient. Similarly, a patient would not be treated for mild hyponatremia of pregnancy. Alternatively, hypovolemia severe enough to result in hyponatremia should be treated with fluid replacement. In cases of hyponatremia associated with impaired water excretion (e.g., SIADH, drug therapy) or decreased effective blood volume with increased total body water (e.g., cirrhosis) the usual treatment is water restriction. An adjunctive approach to water restriction is the use of agents that block the action of ADH at the collecting tubule. Lithium carbonate and demeclocycline are two such agents. Only rarely is a patient treated with hypertonic saline.

DISORDERS OF HYPEROSMOLALITY— THE HYPERNATREMIC PATIENT

In the previous section, the pathogenesis and clinical approach to hyponatremia are discussed. In most, but not all, cases of hyponatremia, there is coexisting hypotonicity. Exceptions include the presence of an unmeasured osmolyte (e.g., glycerol, mannitol) and significant hyperglycemia. Hypernatremia, however, is always associated with hypertonicity.

Hypertonicity can arise in a number of clinical settings. In general, these settings are associated with solute gain, hypotonic fluid loss without free-water replacement, or pure water loss.

Pure solute gain most often occurs when excess sodium salts are administered to a patient, resulting in iatrogenic hypernatremia. This could occur in the setting of a cardiac arrest patient to whom sodium bicarbonate is administered in high concentration to treat the accompanying metabolic acidosis.

Hypertonic fluid losses may be extrarenal or renal in origin. The fluid loss is hypotonic with respect to plasma. Extrarenal fluid loss can occur through excessive sweating or through gastrointestinal losses from vomiting or diarrhea. In these cases, the electrolyte composition of the fluid loss varies, but there is both sodium and water loss. Volume contraction occurs, and the kidney responds appropriately by retaining sodium; therefore, the urinary sodium concentration will be low (<10 mEq/L).

Renal hypotonic fluid losses occur as a result of an osmotic diuresis. When solutes are filtered and not reabsorbed by the tubule, there is obligate water and sodium loss. Solutes commonly associated with an osmotic diuresis include glucose when the filtered glucose concentration exceeds the tubules maximal reabsorptive capacity and mannitol, which is often given to treat cerebral edema or prevent radiocontrast-induced renal injury.

Pure water loss may be extrarenal. The lungs excrete water, and this excretion increases in the setting of hyperventilation and fever. Most often, the pure water loss is of renal origin and is associated with an ADH-related defect. This defect may be due to inadequate production or release of ADH or may be due to an inadequate renal response to ADH. This disorder is generically referred to as *diabetes insipidus*. Insipid means tasteless or saltless; the urine of these patients has a low salt content.

CASE 6

A 25-year-old man is unconscious and admitted to the neurosurgical service following a motor vehicle accident. A computed tomographic scan of the head reveals a basilar skull fracture. Within 4 hours, the patient is noted to have an increased urine output (2.5 L per 8-hour shift). Electrolytes from admission and 24 hours after admission show the following:

	Admission	**24 Hours After Admission**
Sodium	140 mEq/L	155 mEq/L
Potassium	3.8 mEq/L	4.0 mEq/L
Chloride	102 mEq/L	115 mEq/L
Bicarbonate	24 mEq/L	35 mEq/L
BUN	14 mg/dl	30 mg/dl
Creatinine	1.2 mg/dl	1.3 mg/dl
Glucose	80 mg/dl	85 mg/dl

CASE DISCUSSION

This patient has a defect in the production or of the pituitary release of ADH. This disorder is referred to as *central diabetes insipidus*, because this defect arises from a central nervous system disorder. Central diabetes insipidus is also seen in association with tumors, infections (e.g., meningitis, encephalitis, tuberculosis), cerebral aneurysms, and histiocytosis.

Although the role of ADH in water conservation is very important, the thirst response appears to be even more critical. An individual who is able to ingest large quantities of water can generally avoid the development of hypertonicity even in the absence of detectable ADH. Thus, the water loss produces hypertonicity only when there is an associated defect in water intake. Water intake is restricted in an unconscious patient. Water intake can also be restricted in infants, the elderly, or patients who are immobilized.

A defect in ADH activity may occur at the level of the kidney, as illustrated in Case 7.

CASE 7

A 40-year-old man with a 5-year history of bipolar affective disorder visits his psychiatrist with complaints of polyuria, nocturia, and polydipsia. His current therapy includes lithium carbonate, 250 mg, 4 times daily. The following are his plasma electrolytes:

Sodium	150 mEq/L
Potassium	4.0 mEq/L
Chloride	115 mEq/L
Bicarbonate	28 mEq/L
BUN	18 mg/dl
Creatinine	1.5 mg/dl
Glucose	90 mg/dl
Lithium	1.5 mEq/L

CASE DISCUSSION

This patient is mildly hypertonic and polyuric as a result of a lithium-induced defect in ADH action at the level of the renal tubule. Patients with normal circulating levels of ADH who can not raise their urine osmolalities above that of plasma suffer from *nephrogenic diabetes insipidus.* Renal tubular unresponsiveness to ADH can be associated with several disorders, both acquired and congenital. Aside from lithium carbonate, drugs such as demeclocycline, methoxyflurane, and amphotericin B can cause nephrogenic diabetes insipidus. Other conditions associated include hypercalcemia, hypokalemia, and renal interstitial diseases such as sarcoidosis, amyloidosis, sickle cell nephropathy, chronic pyelonephritis, and analgesic nephropathy. Renal tubular unresponsiveness to ADH in these later cases is probably the result of disruption of the medullary interstitial anatomy, which is critical for creation of the osmotic gradient for ADH-dependent antidiuresis.

Most cases of hypertonicity are diagnosed when hypernatremia is detected on an electrolyte panel. The most common patient complaint is polyuria, which occurs at a volume of at least 3 L/day. If the etiology of the polyuria is not apparent in the patient's history, provocative tests are often helpful, as illustrated in Problem 6.

PROBLEM 6

You are a member of the renal consult service and are asked to evaluate 4 patients complaining of polyuria. The attending nephrologist suggests that each patient's water intake be restricted until they each have lost a minimum of 3% of their body weight. Twelve hours later, you are asked to measure their urine osmolality and then administer 5 units of aqueous vasopressin subcutaneously. One hour later, you repeat the urine osmolality measurements. The following values are obtained:

Patient	U_{Osm} After Water Deprivation (mOsm/kg Water)	U_{Osm} After ADH Administration (mOsm/kg Water)	Plasma Sodium (mEq/L)
A	280	no increase	150
B	>500	no increase	130
C	>800	little increase	145
D	250	600	153

Determine the likely cause of the polyuria for each patient.

ANSWER

Patient A probably has nephrogenic diabetes insipidus. He is unable to concentrate his urine after water deprivation and demonstrates no change with the exogenous administration of ADH, consistent with his tubular unresponsiveness.

(continued)

Patient B probably has psychogenic polydipsia. She is able to partially concentrate her urine. However, the loss of her interstitial osmotic gradient contributes to both the inability to maximally concentrate urine and the lack of response to ADH infusion.

Patient C is normal. He concentrates his urine after water deprivation.

Patient D has central diabetes insipidus. She does not concentrate her urine with water deprivation but can respond appropriately to the exogenous infusion of ADH.

As with hypotonicity disorders, the severity of the symptoms associated with hypertonicity depend on both the degree and the rate of development of the hypertonicity. The clinical signs are primarily neurologic and include muscle weakness, lethargy, and twitching. In severe cases, seizures and coma may ensue.

TREATMENT

Hypertonicity results in the movement of water out of cells and down its osmotic gradient. The brain adapts to this loss of water initially by shrinking and then by accumulating osmotically active solutes such as inositol, betaine, and glycerophosphorylcholine. If water is replaced too rapidly in such a patient, then cerebral edema may ensue, resulting in coma, seizures, or even death. Hypernatremia should therefore be reversed slowly, by a rate no greater than 2 mEq/L per hour. The requisite water replacement can be determined by calculating a patient's water deficit. For these calculations, the following is assumed: (1) normal body sodium concentration is 140 mEq/L; (2) total body water is 60% of body weight; (3) sodium distributes through total body water. The latter assumption is obviously false, but it accounts for the loss of water from both intracellular and extracellular compartments.

PROBLEM 7

Calculate the water deficit of an 80-kg man with a serum sodium concentration of 158 mEq/L.

ANSWER

Normal total body water is $80 \times 0.6 = 48$ L.

Normal total body sodium is 48 L $\times 140$ mEq/L $= 6720$ mEq.

Assuming that total body sodium is constant as water is lost, then the total body water of this patient is 6720 mEq/158 mEq/L $= 42.5$ L.

Water deficit is 48 L $- 42.5$ L $= 5.5$ L.

Alternatively, the following formula can be used to calculate the water deficit:

$$\text{Water deficit} = (0.6)(\text{body weight in kg})(1 - 140/P_{Na})$$

SELECTED READING

Feig PV. Hyponatremia and hypertonic syndromes. Med Clin North Am 1981;65:271.

Humes HD. Disorders of water metabolism. In: Koko JP, Tannen RL, eds. Fluids and electrolytes. Philadelphia: WB Saunders, 1986.

Schrier RW. Pathogenesis of sodium and water retention, high-output and low-output cardiac failure, nephrotic syndrome, cirrhosis, and pregnancy. N Engl J Med 1988;319:1065.

Lippincott's Pathophysiology Series: Renal Pathophysiology, edited by James A. Shayman. J. B. Lippincott Company, Philadelphia © 1995.

CHAPTER

2

Sodium

James A. Shayman

OBJECTIVES

By the end of this chapter the reader should be able to:

- Calculate the volume of the body fluid compartments.
- Know the concentrations of the major ions in the intracellular and extra-cellular compartments.
- Understand how water is exchanged between body fluid compartments.
- Understand how Starling's forces control the distribution of fluid across membranes.
- Understand the concepts of glomerular filtration, renal clearance, and fractional excretion.
- Understand the afferent and efferent responses that occur in response to changes in volume.
- Understand elementary structure–function relations between the nephron and sodium transport.
- Understand the role of aldosterone, angiotensin II, catecholamines, and atrial natriuretic factor in regulating volume.
- Understand clinical parameters used in the assessment of a patient's volume status.
- Understand the basic pathophysiology underlying common disorders of volume contraction and volume expansion.

The regulation of the *size* of an individual's fluid volume is critical for life. Sodium and water metabolism are central to fluid regulation. However, the human body has adapted distinct mechanisms for controlling sodium and water homeostasis. Disorders of sodium metabolism are primarily manifested as changes in body volume. In contrast, disorders of water metabolism are primarily manifested as changes in solute concentration or osmolality.

The regulation of volume can be viewed on several levels. Fluid within the body is divided into three major compartments: intracellular, extracellular, and transcellular. The extracellular compartment consists of interstitial and intravascular compartments. The distribution of water between these compartments is the result of the ionic composition of the respective compartments, because in general, water moves freely across membranes, but ionic solutes do not. The clinical assessment of volume depends on measurements of extracellular volume, which is primarily controlled by sodium homeostasis. The regulation of sodium balance is a consequence of physical factors affecting fluid movement across cell membranes, the renal handling of sodium, and several redundant systems that comprise a complex affector and effector network that maintains volume in each fluid compartment.

THE MEASUREMENT OF FLUID COMPARTMENT VOLUMES

Volumes are normally measured directly by pouring the fluid into a graduated vessel. This is impossible if the volume is too large or if the fluid to be measured is not fully retrievable. In these cases, volumes can be measured by dilution. For example, if a dye that can be measured colorimetrically is added to an unknown volume of water, then by measuring the concentration of the dye, the volume of water can be calculated. In other words, if 10 mg of dye is added to a volume of water, and the concentration of dye is measured as 0.01 mg/ml, the volume of water can be calculated as follows:

$$\text{volume} = \text{quantity of dye/concentration of dye}$$
$$= 10 \text{ mg}/0.01 \text{ mg/ml} = 1000 \text{ ml} \qquad [2\text{-}1]$$

The validity of such measurements depends on the assumption that the dye is thoroughly mixed and that it remains in the volume to be measured. Thus, when the same principle is applied to the measurement of fluid compartments in an organism, the volume (or volume of distribution) must be corrected for the excretion and metabolism of the dye or tracer:

$$\text{volume of distribution} = \frac{(\text{quantity administered} - \text{quantity excreted and metabolized})}{\text{concentration}} \qquad [2\text{-}2]$$

PROBLEM 1

The tritiated isotope of water $[^3H]_2O$ is administered to a 90-kg man to quantify total body water. The total loss of $[^3H]_2O$ through urinary and fecal excretion and respiratory losses is 4% of the administered load. The amount of $[^3H]_2O$ incorporated into newly synthesized compounds during the period of infusion and equilibration is negligible. If 10^6 disintegrations per minute (dpm) of $[^3H]_2O$ in 10 ml of saline are given in-

(continued)

travenously, and 19.2 dpm/ml are measured in the plasma of the subject, then what is the volume of body water in this man?

ANSWER

$$(1{,}000{,}000 \text{ dpm} - 40{,}000 \text{ dpm})/19.2 \text{ dpm/ml} = 50{,}000 \text{ ml or } 50 \text{ L}$$

Therefore, because this man weighs 90 kg, body water comprises 50 kg/90 kg, or 55.6% of his body weight.

The determination of total body water with isotopes is cumbersome and not highly accurate. A considerably more practical method for assessing total body water is to measure a patient's weight.

Extracellular volume measurements are more difficult to determine than total body water measurements. No ideal substance exists that is rapidly diffusible across blood vessels, that distributes uniformly within interstitial areas, and that is excluded from intracellular compartments. Markers that have been used for extracellular volume measurements include insulin, sucrose, mannitol, thiocyanate, and thiosulfate. The estimated volumes of distribution using these compounds range widely, from 16% to 23%.

Transcellular fluid is the fraction of the extracellular fluid that includes cerebrospinal, intraocular, pleural, peritoneal, and synovial fluids. These fluid compartments are defined by the property that they are separated from the plasma fluid by both the capillary endothelium and by a specialized layer of epithelial cells.

Plasma volume is more easily measured. It is defined as the volume of distribution of a substance confined to the vascular bed. Albumin labeled with iodine-131 or a dye such as Evans blue is most commonly used for such measurements.

Intracellular fluid volume cannot be measured directly. It is calculated as the difference between total body water and extracellular fluid. Similarly, the *interstitial fluid volume* is calculated as the difference between the extracellular fluid volume and the plasma volume.

Based on the use of these different fluid compartment markers, the normal volumes of distribution of water have been estimated (Fig. 2-1). Total body water comprises 50% to 70% of total body weight. Therefore, the typical 70-kg man has 42 L of total water. Of this 42 L, the volume of intracellular water is 24.5 L, and the volume of interstitial water and the volume of plasma are 11.2 L and 3.1 L, respectively.

HOW WATER IS EXCHANGED BETWEEN COMPARTMENTS

The role of osmolality in the regulation of water distribution across membranes is introduced in Chapter 1. Almost every cell membrane in the body is freely permeable to water but impermeable to most solutes. It is the osmotic gradient of the impermeant solutes that determines the movement of fluid among body fluid compartments.

Five rules regulate the movement of water between extracellular and intracellular fluid compartments:

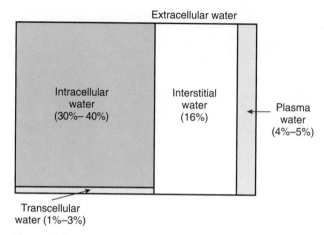

Figure 2-1. Body fluid compartments.

1. Fluid movement between compartments occurs when a membrane permeable to water and impermeable to solute separates two compartments with different concentrations of solutes.
2. Water moves from the compartment with the lower solute concentration into the compartment with the higher solute concentration.
3. Water movement is not affected by membrane-permeable solutes (i.e., ineffective osmoles), such as urea.
4. The impermeable solute concentration gradient determines the magnitude of the water flux.
5. Water movement continues until the solute gradient is equalized or until hydrostatic pressure counterbalances osmotic pressure.

These rules allow prediction of how the osmolar concentrations and volumes of the intracellular and extracellular compartments will change with the addition or removal of fluid or solute.

Consider the effect of ingesting a large volume of pure water (Fig. 2-2A). If a 70-kg man (who is 60% water by weight) rapidly drinks 3 L of water and does not excrete any of the ingested water, then his total body water will increase to 45 L and his intracellular and extracellular osmolality will decrease by 93% (42 L/45 L) to 289 mOsm/kg water. Because water is freely permeable, it diffuses in proportion to the initial intracellular and extracellular volumes. Therefore, extracellular volume increases by (17 L extracellular water/42 L of total water)(3 L) = 1.2 L. By the same reasoning, the intracellular volume increases by 1.8 L. In reality, a water challenge does not change fluid compartments so drastically, because excretion of water begins before all of the water is absorbed.

A much different change in the size and osmolality of intracellular and extracellular fluid compartments occurs with the infusion of a hypertonic solute load (Fig. 2-2B). Suppose a 70-kg man receives an infusion of hypertonic saline (200 ml of 9%, or 615 mOsm). Because compartmental osmolality will be maintained, the osmolality rises to 615 mOsm/42 L, or 15 mOsm/kg water, in both extracellular and intracellular fluid compartments. To compensate, water leaves the intracellular compartment. The 25 L of intracellular fluid at an initial osmolality of 300 mOsm/kg water contain a total of 7500 mOsm of solute. A rise in osmolality to 315 mOsm/kg water requires a final volume of 7500 mOsm/315 mOsm/kg water, or 23.8 kg, a decrease of 1.2 kg.

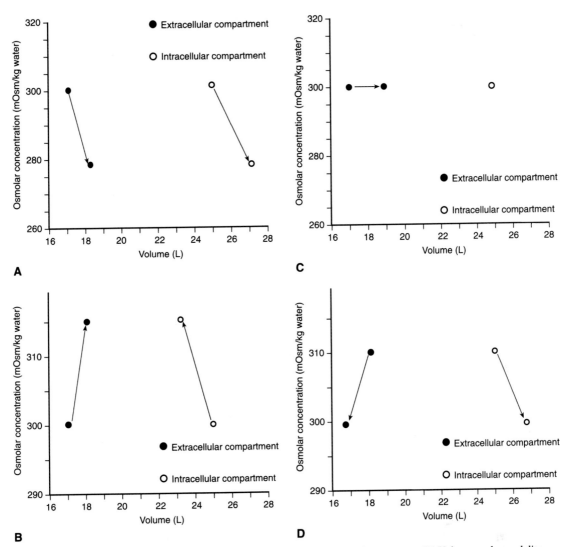

Figure 2-2. (**A**) Volume and osmolality changes associated with ingestion of pure water. (**B**) Volume and osmolality changes associated with infusion of hypertonic saline. (**C**) Volume and osmolality changes associated with infusion of isotonic saline. (**D**) Volume and osmolality changes associated with peritoneal dialysate drainage.

A more practical example is the change in fluid compartments that occurs with the infusion of an isotonic saline solution (Fig. 2-2C). Under these conditions, the extracellular compartment expands in volume without changing the intracellular volume or osmolality or the extracellular osmolality. The saline solution is isotonic, and the sodium chloride remains almost entirely extracellular.

PROBLEM 2

Peritoneal dialysis is one therapeutic option for treating patients with renal failure and removing excess sodium chloride. A 2-L volume of a 4% solution of glucose is infused into the peritoneal cavity of a patient. After 4 hours, 2 L of fluid is drained. During this

(continued)

period, the glucose is absorbed, and the sodium chloride diffuses into the peritoneal space. Predict how the fluid compartment volumes and osmolar concentrations will change.

ANSWER: This case represents an example of the removal of sodium chloride from the extracellular compartment without loss of total body water. The isotonic glucose is transported into the cells and metabolized intracellularly, so that there is no addition of solute to replace the sodium chloride removed in the dialysate. As the dialysate is drained, the extracellular osmolality falls, and water enters the intracellular compartment. Therefore, cellular volume increases at the expense of extracellular volume (Fig. 2-2D).

BODY FLUID COMPOSITION

The ionic compositions of plasma, plasma water, interstitial fluid, and muscle cells are given in Table 2-1.

Because ionic concentrations are expressed as equivalents, electrical neutrality must be maintained. Therefore, within each compartment, the cationic and anionic concentrations are equal. The ionic concentrations of plasma and plasma water are proportionate but not equal. This is because only a fraction of plasma volume (~93%) is water. The remaining volume is occupied by lipid and protein, which occupies a volume that is disproportionate to its contribution to the anionic equivalency. As discussed in Chapter 1, this feature is important in pseudohyponatremic states associated with hyperlipidemia and hyperproteinemia.

Another feature apparent from these ionic composition measurements is the absence of protein in the interstitial compartment. The absence of protein reflects

TABLE 2-1. *FLUID COMPARTMENT ION COMPOSITIONS*

	PLASMA (mEq/L)	PLASMA WATER (mEq/L)	INTERSTITIAL FLUID (mEq/L)	INTRACELLULAR FLUID (mEq/L)
Na^+	142	151	144	10
K^+	4	4.3	4	160
Ca^{+2}	5	5.4	2.5	0
Mg^{+2}	3	3.2	1.5	35
Total cations	154	163.9	152	205
Cl^-	103	109.7	114	2
HCO_3^-	27	28.7	30	8
PO_4^{-2}	2	2.1	2	140
SO_4^{-2}	1	1.1	1	0
Organic acid	5	5.3	5	0
Proteins	16	17	0	55
Total anions	154	163.9	152	205

the special properties of the capillary endothelium, which is effectively imperme-ant to protein but which permits the free diffusion of water and ions from the vas-culature to the interstitial space. Based on the free diffusibility of ions and water across the endothelium, it might be predicted that the ionic concentrations would be equal between these compartments. However, the measured ionic compositions indicate otherwise. This inequality in ionic distribution is explained by the *Gibbs-Donnan rule*. This principle states that if a nondiffusible ion such as a protein is on one side of a membrane that is permeable to other ions, the diffusible ions will dis-tribute unequally on the two sides of the membrane. Three features characterize Gibbs-Donnan equilibrium. The total cation and total anion concentrations on each side of the membrane are equal. The diffusible anion concentration is less on the side of the membrane containing the protein than on the other side of the membrane. The osmotic pressure on the side with the protein is greater than that on the side without the protein. An implication of the third feature of this princi-ple is that fluid should move into the protein containing compartment to offset the inequality in osmotic pressure. In reality, this does not occur, because the hydrosta-tic pressure of plasma opposes the movement of fluid from the interstitial space into the vasculature.

PROBLEM 3

One mOsm/kg water exerts an osmotic effect equivalent to 17 mm Hg. Calculate the os-motic pressure contributed by the diffusible ions (i.e., crystalloids) in the extracellular fluids of a man with normal serum osmolality (300 mOsm/kg water), and contrast that to the osmotic pressure exerted by plasma proteins (i.e., colloids). Assume a contribu-tion by plasma proteins of 1.65 mOsm/kg water.

ANSWER: The total osmotic pressure exerted by crystalloids in the extracellular fluid is:

$$(300 \text{ mOsm/kg water}) \times 17 \text{ mm Hg/mOsm} = 5100 \text{ mm Hg}$$

The total osmotic pressure exerted by proteins in the plasma is:

$$(1.65 \text{ mOsm/kg water}) \times 17 \text{ mm Hg/mOsm} = 28 \text{ mm Hg}$$

The colloid osmotic pressure appears to be trivial in comparison to the crys-talloid oncotic pressure. However, the physiologic effect of the colloid osmotic pressure, or oncotic pressure, is highly significant. The significance lies in the fact that the capillary endothelium is highly permeable to both water and small solutes. Therefore, these small solutes exert no effective osmotic force on the endothe-lium. In contrast, because the protein concentration of the interstium is low, and because proteins do not diffuse across the endothelium, the full osmotic force of these colloids is exerted on the endothelial wall.

STARLING'S FORCES

The distribution of fluid between the vascular and interstitial compartments can be explained on the basis of the hydrostatic and colloid osmotic pressures in the capillaries (Fig. 2-3). This model was first outlined by Starling almost 100 years

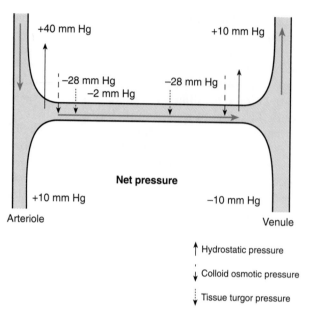

Figure 2-3. Effect of Starling's forces on the fluid distribution between vascular and interstitial fluid compartments.

ago. Blood enters capillaries at a pressure of about 40 mm Hg and promotes the movement of fluid across the capillary endothelium into the interstitial space. As discussed previously, this hydrostatic pressure is opposed by a plasma oncotic pressure of about 28 mm Hg. In addition, an opposing pressure of 2 to 5 mm Hg is exerted by the turgor of the interstitial compartment. Thus, at the beginning of the capillary there is a net pressure of about 10 mm Hg promoting the movement of fluid from the capillary space into the interstitial space. By the end of the capillary, a fall in intravascular pressure has occurred, so that the hydrostatic pressure may be 10 to 15 mm Hg. Thus, there is a net inward pressure of 10 to 15 mm Hg by the time blood has reached the end of the capillary. The algebraic sum of the opposing hydrostatic and colloid osmotic or oncotic pressures is termed the *net filtration pressure.*

GLOMERULAR FILTRATION

Filtration across a capillary membrane not only depends on the net filtration pressure but also on the permeability of the membrane (i.e., hydraulic permeability) and the surface area available for filtration. The product of hydraulic permeability and surface area is termed the filtration coefficient (K_f). The filtration rate (FR) can be expressed by the following equation:

$$FR = \text{hydraulic permeability} \times \text{surface area} \times \text{net filtration pressure}$$

[2-3]

or

$$FR = K_f \times \text{net filtration pressure}$$

In Bowman's capsule, the glomerular equivalent to the interstitial space, the protein content is essentially zero. Therefore, net filtration pressure (NFP) equals the opposing forces of the glomerular capillary pressure (P_{GC}), Bowman's capsule pressure (P_{BC}), and glomerular capillary oncotic pressure (π_{GC}):

$$NFP = P_{GC} - P_{BC} - \pi_{GC} \qquad [2\text{-}4]$$

The filtration rate across the glomerular capillary, or *glomerular filtration rate* (GFR) can therefore be expressed as follows:

$$GRF = K_f \times (P_{GC} - P_{BC} - \pi_{GC}) \qquad [2\text{-}5]$$

As plasma moves through the glomerular capillary, the glomerular capillary pressure falls slightly, and the glomerular capillary oncotic pressure rises, because the concentration of unfiltered colloid increases as water and crystalloids are filtered. The degree of rise in π_{GC} depends on the renal plasma flow. The lower the flow, the greater the rise in π_{GC} that occurs by the end of the glomerular capillary. The result of these changes in π_{GC} and P_{GC} is an overall decrease in net filtration pressure by the end of the glomerular capillary. This relation is shown in Figure 2-4.

Under normal conditions, the total daily net filtration of fluid across all of the capillary membranes in the body, excluding those in the kidney, is 4 L. This fluid is returned to the central circulation via the lymphatic system. In contrast, the GFR is 180 L/day, or 50 to 60 times the plasma volume. The net filtration pressure across glomerular capillaries varies between 10 and 24 mm Hg. The difference in filtration is attributable to a markedly greater filtration coefficient in glomerular capillaries. The greater glomerular capillary filtration is the result of a larger glomerular capillary surface area and a significantly greater hydraulic permeability.

The GFR is constantly changing, because many factors can affect K_f, P_{GC}, P_{BC}, and π_{GC} in both healthy and diseased patients. The glomerular capillary surface area may decrease with the contraction of the smooth muscle, as in glomerular mesangial cells. K_f, and in turn GFR, may fall under conditions in which mesangial cell contraction is stimulated. P_{GC} changes in response to three factors: renal

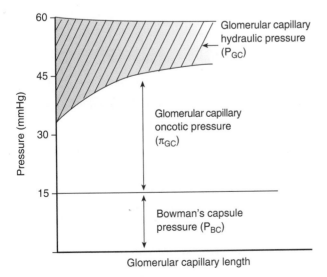

Figure 2-4. Net filtration pressure across the glomerular capillary is denoted by the shaded area of the graph.

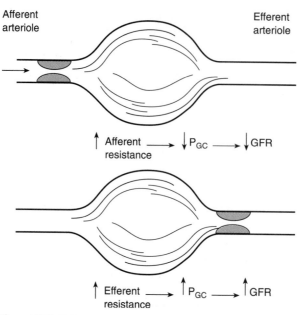

Figure 2-5. Relation among afferent and efferent arteriolar resistances, glomerular capillary pressure (P_{GC}) and glomerular filtration rate (GFR).

arterial pressure, afferent, arteriolar resistance, and efferent arteriolar resistance (Fig. 2-5). An increase in afferent resistance will decrease P_{GC}; conversely, an increase in efferent arteriolar resistance will increase P_{GC}. Contraction of the efferent arteriole and increases in efferent arteriolar resistance are particularly sensitive to the hormone angiotensin II. An increase in renal plasma flow under conditions of constant P_{GC} tends to decrease π_{GC} because of a slower increase in the colloid concentration in the glomerular capillary. The physiologic factors that influence GFR are listed in Table 2-2.

TABLE 2-2. *PHYSIOLOGIC FACTORS INFLUENCING GLOMERULAR FILTRATION RATE (GFR)*

DETERMINANTS OF GFR	PHYSIOLOGIC FACTORS
Filtration coefficient (K_f)	Glomerular capillary surface area (mesangial cell relaxation increases, contraction decreases K_f and GFR)
Glomerular capillary pressure (P_{GC})	Renal arterial pressure, afferent and efferent arteriolar resistances (increases arterial pressure, decreased afferent arteriolar resistance and increased efferent arteriolar resistance increase GFR)
Glomerular capillary oncotic pressure (π_{GC})	Systemic plasma colloid concentration and renal plasma flow (increased plasma colloids decrease, and decreased plasma flow will increase π_{GC} and decrease GFR)

PROBLEM 4

For each clinical disorder, predict the response in GFR.

   A. *Early diabetes mellitus associated with glomerular hypertrophy, mesangial cell relaxation, and preglomerular afferent vasodilatation.*
   B. *Late diabetic nephropathy with mesangial matrix deposition and glomerular basement membrane thickening.*
   C. *Waldenström's macroglobuminemia with a plasma concentration of IgM antibody of 4 g/dl.*
   D. *Obstructive uropathy caused by benign prostatic hyperplasia.*

ANSWERS

   A. During the early phases of diabetes mellitus (i.e., the first 5 years following onset) the GFR is significantly increased. The exact mechanism for the hyperfiltration is unknown; however, the increased glomerular capillary surface area as a result of glomerular capillary growth and mesangial cell relaxation, and increased plasma flow rate as a result of decreased afferent arteriolar resistance are probably significant determinants of the increased filtration rate. Thus, both increased K_f and P_{GC} probably contribute to the increased filtration rate.
   B. Long-standing diabetes (i.e., of 10 years or longer) is most commonly associated with pathologic findings of mesangial matrix expansion with deposition of extracellular matrix within the mesangial space and basement membrane thickening. Thus, a decrease in K_f is probably the major cause of the fall in GFR.
   C. The increase in monoclonal IgM accompanying this plasma cell dyscrasia will raise P_{GC} and therefore decrease GFR.
   D. Obstructive uropathy will decrease GFR as a result of an increase in P_{BC}. Vasoconstrictive prostaglandins such as thromboxane A_2 probably also contribute to the decrease in GFR by decreasing both K_f and P_{GC} as a result of afferent arteriolar constriction and mesangial cell contraction.

TUBULAR REABSORPTION AND FRACTIONAL EXCRETION

PROBLEM 5

As stated previously, the average person filters 180 L of plasma per day. If sodium, urea, and glucose are freely filtered from the glomerular capillary to Bowman's space, calculate the amount of these substances filtered per day. The molecular weight of sodium is 23, and the concentrations of urea and glucose are 14 mg/dl and 100 mg/dl, respectively.

(continued)

> **ANSWER:** The filtered load of sodium is:
>
> $$(23 \text{ mg/mEq})(151 \text{ mEq/L})(180 \text{ L/day})(1 \text{ g/1000 mg})$$
> $$= 6.25 \text{ g/day}$$
>
> The filtered load of glucose is:
>
> $$(100 \text{ mg/dl})(10 \text{ dl/L})(180 \text{ L/day})(1 \text{ g/1000 mg})$$
> $$= 180 \text{ g/day}$$
>
> The filtered load of urea is:
>
> $$(14 \text{ mg/dl})(10 \text{ dl/L})(180 \text{ L/day})(1 \text{ g/1000 mg}) = 25.2 \text{ g/day}$$

A typical person can excrete only 3 g of sodium per day. Therefore, more than 99.5% of all the filtered sodium is reabsorbed. Glucose is even more efficiently reabsorbed. A healthy person without diabetes mellitus does not excrete any detectable glucose. In contrast, the waste product urea is less efficiently reabsorbed. About 50% of the filtered urea, approximately 12 g, is excreted per day, indicating that the kidney is highly selective in the substances that are reabsorbed following filtration.

In general, the filtered quantities of water and filtered plasma substances are impressively large. The 70-kg man whose total body water equals 42 kg filters 4.5 times his body total water volume or 40 times his plasma volume each day.

As discussed in Chapter 1, the kidney is the effector organ for the control of water metabolism, and the reabsorption of water is highly regulated. Similarly, the reabsorption of filtered sodium, as well as other ions, is highly controlled. In contrast, under normal conditions, the regulation of plasma glucose concentration is not regulated by the kidney. The tubular reabsorption is so great that the kidney acts as if no glucose was filtered. However, under conditions of high glucose (e.g., diabetes mellitus) the tubule's ability to reabsorb the filtered glucose is exceeded, and the kidney plays an important role in lowering plasma glucose.

Sodium balance is the most important determinant of body volume, and the kidney is the most important effector in the regulation of sodium balance. An average person may vary their sodium intake significantly on a daily basis. Sodium chloride intake may be as little as 50 mg/day or as great as 20 g/day. For a typical daily intake of 10 g of sodium chloride, only 0.5 is lost through sweating and intestinal excretion. The majority of the sodium chloride balance is maintained by renal excretion.

Without much consideration, it is evident that there is a daily net excretion of sodium, but that this excretion represents only a small fraction of the total filtered sodium. The net excretion of any compound may represent the balance between secretion and reabsorption. But without any knowledge of how sodium is handled in the nephron, it is still possible to quantify the net secretion and reabsorption that is occurring. This value is expressed as the mass of filtered sodium that is excreted, or as the *fractional excretion of sodium.*

The fractional excretion of a compound X is derived as follows:

$$\text{fraction excretion of X} = \frac{\text{mass X secreted}}{\text{mass X filtered}} \qquad [2\text{-}6]$$

$$\text{mass of X excreted} = \text{the urinary concentration of X } (U_X) \\ \times \text{ urinary volume } (V) \qquad [2\text{-}7]$$

$$\text{mass of X filtered} = \text{GFR} \times \text{plasma concentration of X } (P_X) \qquad [2\text{-}8]$$

or

$$(FE_X) = (U_X)(V)/(GFR)(P_X) \qquad [2\text{-}9]$$

As discussed in Chapter 1, the clearance of creatinine is a close approximation of GFR. Since $GFR = (U_{Cr})(V)(P_{Cr})$, substitution of these values eliminates the need to measure urine volume:

$$(FE_X) = (U_X)(P_{Cr})(V)/(U_{Cr})(P_X)(V) = (U_X)(P_{Cr})/(U_{Cr})(P_X) \qquad [2\text{-}10]$$

Thus, simply knowing the urinary and plasma concentrations of creatinine and the compound of interest allows calculation of the fractional excretion of that compound.

PROBLEM 6

Calculate the fractional excretion of sodium for a patient with the following values:

Plasma sodium	140 mEq/L
Urinary sodium	20 mEq/L
Plasma creatinine	1 mg/dl
Urinary creatinine	15 mg/dl

ANSWER: FENa = (20 mEq/L)(1 mg/dl)/(140 mEq/L)(15 mg/dl) = 0.0095, or approximately 1%. This patient excretes only 1% of the total sodium filtered by his kidneys. Under conditions of excess sodium intake, his FENa may increase to 5%. Under conditions of decreased sodium intake, his FENa may decrease to 0.1%. The measurement of FENa is often a good clinical indicator of the presence of a physiologic stimulus for the retention of sodium by the kidney. The clinical use of FENa is discussed later in this chapter.

SODIUM HANDLING IN THE KIDNEY: STRUCTURE–FUNCTION RELATIONS

The handling of sodium by the kidney is highly efficient, tightly regulated, and controlled by a variety of factors, both intrinsic and extrinsic to the kidney. Once filtered, sodium must move from the lumen of the tubule to the renal interstitium in a vectorial manner. This is possible because the tubular epithelial cells are polarized and maintain distinct transporters on the basolateral and apical membranes. The physical and functional separation of basolateral and apical domains is possible because of the presence of tight junctions. Tight junctions can be visualized as being similar to the plastic holder around a six pack of beer. The apical side is analogous to the top of the cans; the basolateral membranes are analogous to the bottom and sides of the cans (Fig. 2-6).

There are only two routes for solutes and water to move across the tubular epithelia. One route, the transcellular route, is through cells. The other route, the paracellular route, is between cells. The driving forces for sodium movement from the lumen to the interstitium include the concentration gradient and the electrical potential. These gradients are developed by the energy requiring Na^+,K^+-ATPase transporters located on the basolateral surfaces of the epithelia throughout the nephron. For each molecule of ATP used by this enzyme, three Na^+ are pumped out of the cell, and two K^+ are transported inwardly. Two important consequences occur as a result of the NA^+,K^+-ATPase. A chemical gradient for Na^+ is created favoring the movement of Na^+ into the epithelia. An electrical gradient is created, because three cations are transported outward for every two K^+ transported inwardly. K^+ leakage across the membrane lowers the membrane potential, making the inside of the tubular membrane negative compared with the outside of the membrane (see Chap. 3).

Sodium and potassium are thus transported across the basolateral membrane uphill through a *primary active transport* process. The potential energy stored as a result of this electrochemical gradient provides the energy needed for Na^+ transport throughout the nephron. Using this potential energy, the tubular epithelia can transport sodium across the apical membrane by way of three primary mechanisms. The first mechanism is downhill movement through a sodium channel. The electrochemical gradient promotes the movement of sodium by diffusion through a membrane pore that is relatively specific for sodium.

The second and third mechanisms occur through *secondary active transport* processes. A cotransporter may move sodium and a second substance using a symporter. In this case, the other substance is transported against an electrical or concentration gradient using the potential energy stored in the form of the electrochemical gradient for sodium. The coupled movement of sodium and glucose in the proximal tubule is an example of secondary active cotransport. A substance

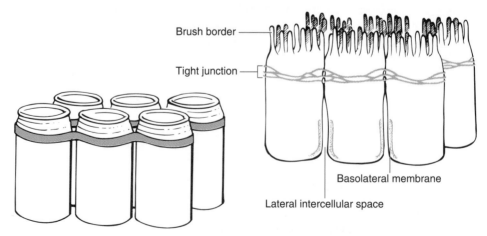

Brush border

Tight junction

Basolateral membrane

Lateral intercellular space

Figure 2-6. Comparison between transporting renal epithelia and a six-pack of beer.

may move out of a cell as sodium moves into a cell against an electrochemical gradient. In this case, the *countertransport* occurs by way of an *antiporter* in a secondary active transport process. The coupled movement of protons into the proximal tubular lumen via the Na^+, H^+ antiporter is an example of this process.

Approximately 70% of the total sodium filtered is reabsorbed in the proximal tubule. Reabsorption occurs through both cotransport and countertransport mechanisms. In addition, a large amount of sodium and water are reabsorbed paracellularly across permeable junctional complexes. The intraluminal fluid remains isoosmotic throughout the proximal tubule; however, the major solutes are not transported to an equal extent (Fig. 2-7). Glucose and amino acids are almost totally reabsorbed by the end of the tubule. Seventy-five to eighty percent of the bicarbonate is reclaimed. These changes occur while only about 50% of the filtered volume is reabsorbed.

The luminal transporters responsible for proximal tubule sodium transport are primarily sodium–glucose, sodium–amino acid, sodium–organic anion, and sodium–phosphate symporters and sodium–proton antiporters. As stated previously, basolateral transport of sodium occurs by way of the Na^+,K^+-ATPase (Fig. 2-8). Because bicarbonate, phosphate, and organic anions are actively transported, the chloride concentration increases as filtrate moves down the proximal tubule. As the chloride concentration rises in excess of the blood chloride concentration, a chemical gradient is created favoring the movement of chloride through cellular transporters and paracellularly. The movement of chloride creates a lumen-positive potential favoring the paracellular movement of additional sodium.

In Chapter 1, the transport characteristics of the loop of Henle are discussed. The thin descending and ascending limbs of Henle's loop transport water and sodium passively. The thin descending limb is permeable to water but not to solutes; the thin ascending limb is highly permeable to solutes but not to water.

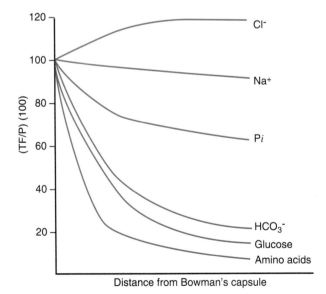

Figure 2-7. Proximal tubular fluid composition as a function of proximal tubule length. TF/P, tubular fluid to plasma concentration; Pi, inorganic phosphate. (Redrawn from Rector FC. Am J Physiol 1983;249:F461.)

Lumen   Interstitium

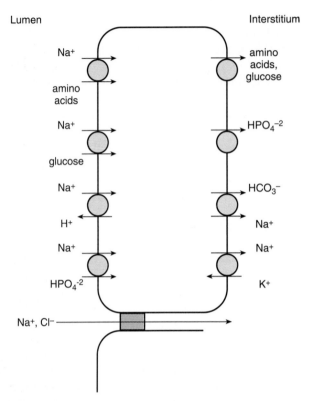

Figure 2-8. Transport characteristics of the proximal tubular epithelium.

The consequence of these solubility differences is the formation of a solute-rich, concentrated urine by the tip of Henle's loop and an increasingly more dilute urine as filtrate reaches the thick ascending limb.

The thick ascending limb is effectively impermeant to water. Sodium is reabsorbed across the apical membrane by way of a cotransporter that couples the movement of 1 Na^+ and 1 K^+ ion with 2 Cl^- ions. This secondary active transport process is driven by the basolateral Na^+,K^+-ATPase. K^+ recycles across the apical membrane through apical K^+ channels. This promotes sodium uptake in two ways. K^+ is present in a concentration sufficient to allow continued transport of sodium by the cotransporter. The movement of K^+ from the thick ascending limb cell into the lumen creates a lumen-positive potential that promotes the transport of additional sodium through paracellular routes.

Sodium transport in the distal tubule occurs primarily by way of an apical transporter that couples sodium and chloride. Energy is provided by the Na^+,K^+-ATPase. Two types of cells are present in the cortical collecting duct: principal cells and intercalated cells. The intercalated cells have a primary role in urine acidification. The principal cells control most of the sodium transport in this segment. These cells have apical sodium channels. Sodium transport is promoted by the electrochemical gradient created by the basolateral Na^+,K^+-ATPase. The transport of sodium across the principal cells creates a lumen-negative potential that promotes the transport of chloride.

THE REGULATION OF RENAL SODIUM REABSORPTION

GFR is a key determinant in renal sodium excretion, because the amount of sodium filtered across the glomerulus is directly proportionate to the GFR. Only a small change in GFR is required to induce a massive change in sodium excretion, as demonstrated in Problem 7.

PROBLEM 7

Calculate the change in filtered sodium that would occur over 1 day resulting from an increase in GFR from 120 ml/minute to 125 ml/minute.

ANSWER

$$(140 \text{ mEq/L})(0.125 - 0.120 \text{ L/minute})(1440 \text{ minute/day})$$
$$= 1008 \text{ mEq Na/day}$$

If a person excreted an isoosmotic urine, then an increase in sodium excretion of 1000 mEq/day (or 2000 mEq of NaCl) would result in an increased urine output of 6.66 L/day. In other words, a trivial change in GFR would result in a massive change in urine output.

Because GFR does vary, there must exist alternative mechanisms for regulating renal sodium excretion. In fact, multiple factors contribute to the renal regulation of sodium balance. These factors may be thought of as those that are either extrinsic or intrinsic to the kidney. An example of an extrinsic factor is a circulating hormone or humoral factor that increases or decreases sodium excretion. An intrinsic factor is an intrarenal physical property that regulates sodium handling independent of any extrinsic influence.

It has been demonstrated experimentally that an increase or decrease in GFR is associated with a respective increase or decrease in sodium reabsorption. The association between filtration and tubular reabsorption is referred to as *glomerulotubular balance.* There are at least two physical factors that contribute to glomerulotubular balance. Peritubular Starling's forces may promote increased sodium reabsorption in the setting of increased glomerular filtration. After filtration occurs at the glomerulus, blood leaves the glomerulus through the efferent arteriole and progresses to the peritubular capillaries. The greater the degree of filtration, the greater the protein concentration in the peritubular capillary, and the greater the oncotic pressure. The increased oncotic pressure exerts a greater force in the promotion of fluid from the tubular interstitium. Because the proximal tubule is a leaky epithelium, the increase in peritubular fluid uptake promotes increased transport of sodium and water across the proximal tubule.

A second factor contributing to glomerulotubular balance is the change in composition of the proximal tubule filtrate. Under conditions of increased glomerular filtration, there is an increased delivery of glucose, amino acids, phosphate, and organic ions to the proximal tubule. Because sodium is cotransported with these compounds, if the tubular capacity (Tm) for the reabsorption of these solutes is not exceeded, increased filtration will result in increased reabsorption of sodium. The net effect of both changes in peritubular oncotic pressure and proximal tubule solute delivery is to dampen changes in sodium excretion following changes in GFR.

Several extrinsic factors regulate sodium handling by the kidney. *Atrial natriuretic factor* (ANF) is released from cardiac atria following stretch and induces an increase in sodium excretion by two mechanisms. ANF increases GFR and inhibits sodium reabsorption in the medullary collecting duct. Another natriuretic compound is *ouabain*. This low-molecular-weight compound is produced in the hypothalamus, circulates through the bloodstream, and inhibits Na^+,K^+-ATPase in the kidney and elsewhere. Other agents identified as potential regulators of sodium excretion include corticosteroids, estrogens, growth hormone, and insulin, which enhance reabsorption, and progesterone, parathyroid hormone, and glucagon, which decrease sodium reabsorption. Intrarenal factors that are formed within and act locally (i.e., autocoids) include dopamine, kinins, and prostaglandins.

The most important extrarenal factor regulating sodium reabsorption by the kidney is *aldosterone.* This steroid is synthesized in the zona glomerulosa in the cortex of the adrenal gland. On a quantitative basis, aldosterone regulates the reabsorption of approximately 2% of the total filtered sodium. It acts on the principal cells of the cortical collecting duct, a point in the nephron where 90% of the filtered sodium has already been reabsorbed.

Aldosterone binds to intracellular receptors and is translocated to the cell nucleus, where it stimulates gene transcription. The proteins that are subsequently synthesized mediate the opening of sodium channels in the apical membrane. Increased sodium enters the principal cells and stimulates the activity of the basolateral Na^+,K^+-ATPase. The increased transport of potassium into the cell across the basolateral membrane results in increased K^+ secretion as K^+ exits through luminal potassium channels.

Aldosterone secretion can be regulated by the plasma sodium concentration, the plasma potassium concentration, and the pituitary hormone adrenocorticotropic hormone (ACTH), factors that are independent of the kidney. However, aldosterone's most important action is as the effector arm of a hormonal axis involved in the correction of perturbations in extracellular volume. This axis consists of renin, angiotensin II, and aldosterone.

THE RENIN–ANGIOTENSIN II–ALDOSTERONE AXIS

The biochemical relation among renin, angiotensin II, and aldosterone are shown in Figure 2-9. Renin is a proteolytic enzyme stored and secreted by the granular cells of the juxtaglomerular apparatus. The substrate for this enzyme is an-

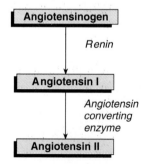

Figure 2-9. Pathway for angiotensin II formation.

TABLE 2-3.	*PHYSIOLOGIC EFFECTS OF ANGIOTENSIN II*
Renal	Directly stimulates Na reabsorption in the proximal tubule
	Decreases glomerular filtration rate by glomerular arteriolar constriction
Central nervous system	Facilitates sympathetic activity
	Increases antidiuretic hormone secretion
	Increases thirst response
Vascular	Stimulates vascular smooth muscle contraction resulting in increased arteriolar constriction
Adrenal	Stimulates aldosterone secretion

giotensinogen, a protein formed in the liver that circulates through the plasma. Renin splits this peptide, forming a 10-amino-acid peptide known as angiotensin I. A second enzyme, angiotensin converting enzyme, cleaves the terminal two amino acids, forming angiotensin II.

Angiotensin II exerts numerous biologic effects. Most of these effects result in the elevation and maintenance of blood pressure. Angiotensin II accomplishes these effects by increasing sodium and water retention and by increasing the resistance of the vasculature. These effects are summarized in Table 2-3.

Although renin can be produced at sites other than the kidney (e.g., brain, uterus), it is the release of renin from the kidney in response to changes in extracellular volume that regulates the formation of angiotensin II and aldosterone. The sensing and effector site for renin release is the *juxtaglomerular apparatus* (JGA). The JGA consists of three primary types of cells: the renin-secreting granular cells, the glomerular mesangial cells, and the tubular macula densa cells (Fig. 2-10). The macula densa is contiguous with both the mesangial cell compartment and the renin secreting granular cells. Under conditions of increased volume, sodium and chloride delivery to the distal tubule are increased. NaCl reabsorption in the distal tubule is likewise increased, and this provides a signal to inhibit renin release. Under conditions of volume contraction, NaCl delivery is decreased, and renin secretion is increased. This signaling–effector system permits the kidney to regulate sodium reabsorption and vascular contraction at the level of the individual nephron.

Other factors regulating renin secretion include renal sympathetic nerves, which stimulate renin release through β_1-adrenergic receptors, and angiotensin II, which inhibits renin secretion. Angiotensin II, formed indirectly by renin release, is one limb of a negative feedback loop. In addition, the granular cells themselves may act as baroreceptors. When stretched, the granular cells release less renin.

AFFERENT RESPONSES TO CHANGES IN VOLUME

The pivotal contribution of the kidneys to the afferent and efferent limbs of volume regulation has been considered. However, it is important to maintain a less renocentric approach to volume regulation, because multiple other sites of the afferent limb in volume regulation are present throughout the body.

Intrathoracic volume receptors are present in both the cardiac atria and pul-

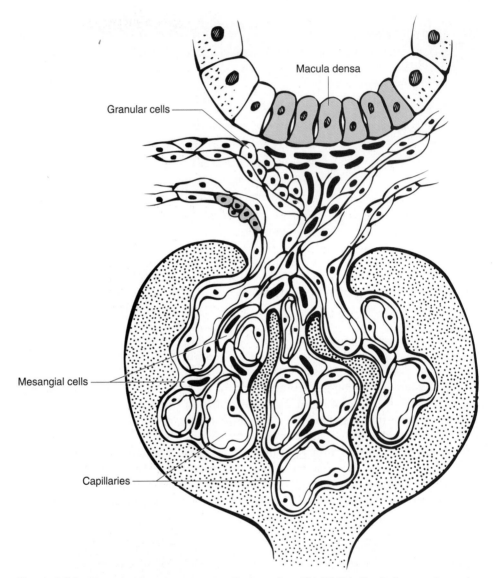

Macula densa

Granular cells

Mesangial cells

Capillaries

Figure 2-10. The juxtaglomerular apparatus. (Redrawn from Kriz W, Kaissling B. Structural organization of the mammalian kidney. In Seldin DW, Giebisch G, eds. The kidney: physiology and pathophysiology. New York: Raven Press, 1985.)

monary veins. Experimentally, distending the cardiac atrium in an animal results in a prompt salt and water diuresis. This response is the result of neural afferent activity transmitted through the vagal nerve to the cardiovascular centers within the medulla. The medulla responds by decreasing the renal adrenergic neural activity, and the result is a decrease in renin release.

The cardiac atria are also endocrine glands. Atrial stretch causes the release of the natriuretic hormone ANF. ANF stimulates sodium excretion by the kidney through several mechanisms. ANF increases GFR by decreasing afferent arteriolar resistance. ANF also decreases tubular sodium reabsorption independent of changes in GFR. In addition, ANF promotes natriuresis by inhibiting renal renin release and adrenal aldosterone synthesis.

Volume receptors also exist in the aortic arch and carotid sinus. Distention of these vascular structures decreases peripheral vascular resistance through a medullary reflex pathway. A reflex arch may also exist between these structures and the kidney. Increased stretch of these structures results in sodium excretion. The liver and kidney themselves may act as volume receptors. These organs are encapsulated. Increasing the interstitial hydrostatic pressure in these organs by a variety of maneuvers results in increased sodium excretion.

DISORDERS OF EXTRACELLULAR VOLUME CONTRACTION

Contraction of the extracellular volume is, by definition, loss of sodium and water in excess of intake. In most cases, the total body volume is decreased in proportion to the decrease in extracellular volume. In other cases, extracellular fluid moves into a third space, such as the peritoneal cavity, resulting in extracellular volume contraction in the setting of euvolemia. Consider Case 1.

CASE 1

A 30-year-old man visits his internist with a 3-day history of fever, chills, crampy abdominal pain, and bloody diarrhea (6–8 bowel movements per day). Over the last 12 hours, he has become progressively weaker and more unsteady with ambulation.

On examination he is pale and appears ill. Vital signs reveal an oral temperature of 38.5°C, respiratory rate of 12 breaths/minute, pulse rate of 100 bpm, and supine blood pressure of 130/70 mm Hg. Upon standing, his pulse increases to 120 bpm and his blood pressure falls to 105/60 mm Hg. His skin turgor is poor, and the oropharynx reveals dry mucous membranes. His intraocular pressure is decreased. There is no axillary sweat. The jugular veins are not visualized. Cardiac examination reveals a tachycardic but regular rate with an increased first heart sound. His laboratory values are as follows:

Sodium	140 mEq/L
Chloride	116 mEq/L
Glucose	70 mg/dl
Potassium	4.0 mEq/L
Bicarbonate	14 mEq/L
Blood urea nitrogen	40 mg/dl
Hemoglobin	10.1 g/dl
Hematocrit	32%
Creatinine	1.2 mg/dl

CASE DISCUSSION

This patient suffers from infectious hemorrhagic diarrhea. His has an extracellular volume deficit due to both blood loss and diarrhea. This patient demonstrates several of the signs and symptoms of extracellular volume contraction resulting from his gastrointestinal losses. The loss of extracellular volume is manifest as changes in intravascular, interstitial, and transcellular fluid compartments.

The changes in blood pressure and pulse rate are sensitive measures of intravascular volume loss. With moderate volume depletion, heart rate and blood pressure may be within normal limits. However, upon standing, there is an *orthostatic* fall in blood pressure accompanied by a rise in heart rate. With severe volume depletion, hypotension and shock may be present. Quantitatively, a drop of more than 15 mm Hg in systolic blood pressure and a rise in pulse rate of more than 15 bpm are considered consistent with mild-to-moderate volume depletion. A decrease in jugular venous pressure is also a helpful finding for establishing the diagnosis of volume depletion.

A decrease in the volume of the interstitial fluid compartment is seen as a loss of skin turgor with tenting of the skin. Transcellular fluid compartment loss can be seen as dryness of the mucous membranes and a decrease in intraocular pressure.

The laboratory data are consistent with both the diarrhea and the patient's response to volume depletion. The hemoglobin and hematocrit reflect the blood loss. The acidosis (see Chap. 4) reflects the loss of bicarbonate in the diarrhea. The increase in both blood urea nitrogen (BUN) and creatinine reflect the decrease in blood flow to the kidney. The proportionately greater increase in BUN reflects the increased reabsorption of urea in response to volume depletion.

The physical findings associated with extracellular volume depletion are listed in Table 2-4.

The source of extracellular fluid loss is obvious in this patient, hemorrhage and diarrhea are easily diagnosed. Often, the source of extracellular fluid loss is not apparent, as seen in Case 2.

CASE 2

A 45-year-old woman arrives at the emergency department with a 3-day history of fever, abdominal pain, and jaundice. Although she has been unable to eat solid foods, her fluid intake has been maintained. She describes a right upper quadrant pain that initially occurred following meals but is now persis-

TABLE 2-4. *PHYSICAL FINDINGS WITH EXTRACELLULAR VOLUME DEPLETION*

FLUID COMPARTMENT	PHYSICAL FINDINGS
Intravascular	Orthostatic fall in systolic blood pressure greater than 15 mm Hg
	Orthostatic rise in pulse rate greater than 15 bpm
	Hypotension while recumbent
Interstitial	Decreased skin turgor
Transcellular	Dry mouth and mucous membranes; decreased intraocular pressure

tent. There is also a sharp, midline pain that radiates to her back. She denies vomiting or diarrhea. On physical examination, she is an ill-appearing woman in moderate distress. Her weight is 50 kg (normal weight is 51 kg), her blood pressure and pulse rate are 120/70 mm Hg and 90 bpm while lying and 105/60 mm Hg and 125 bpm while standing. Her skin and sclera are yellow. Her mucous membranes are dry. Abdominal examination is significant for punch tenderness over the right upper quadrant.

Laboratory data are significant for a total bilirubin of 6.5 mg/dl (normal, 0.25–1.5 mg/dl), amylase of 250 IU/L (normal, 23–85 IU/L) and lipase of 100 IU/dl (normal, 4–24 IU/dl). Abdominal ultrasonography reveals numerous gallstones with biliary ductal dilation. Ascites is also noted.

CASE DISCUSSION

This patient suffers from extracellular fluid loss with orthostatic hypotension. Unlike the first case, however, her total body volume is close to normal, as indicated by her weight. In this case, the extracellular fluid has entered a transcellular compartment, the peritoneal cavity. The basis for her clinical problems are biliary obstruction due to cholelithiasis and pancreatitis resulting from a common biliary duct obstruction. Fluid has entered a third space, and her intravascular volume is diminished.

Volume contraction as a result of loss of intravascular volume into a third space is commonly associated with intestinal obstruction, crush injuries, and pancreatitis.

DISORDERS OF EXTRACELLULAR VOLUME EXPANSION

The clinical definition of extracellular volume expansion is a state of excessive volume overload associated with edema formation. Edema is the accumulation of fluid within an interstitial space such as the feet or the pulmonary interstitium. The most common example of extracellular volume overload is exemplified in the Case 3.

CASE 3

A 65-year-old man with a history of angina and two documented myocardial infarctions visits his physician with a history of progressively increasing shortness of breath and pedal swelling. He reports a decrease in exercise tolerance, with the inability to ascend one flight of stairs and the inability to lie flat in bed without becoming short of breath. On physical examination, his respiratory rate is 24 breaths/minute, blood pressure is 170/95 mm Hg while sitting, and pulse rate is 90 bpm and regular. The patient's weight is 95 kg; his normal weight is 81 kg. His cardiac examination reveals jugular venous distention to 8 cm above the clavicle, a substernal lift, and point of maximal impulse at the left axillary line 5 cm in diameter. The carotid upstroke and amplitude are diminished. In addition, the liver is enlarged, and on application of gentle pressure, there is increased distention of the jugular veins. Pulmonary examination is significant for crackles (rales) extending halfway up the back. His extremities reveal marked pitting edema to the knees. His urinary sodium concentration is 5 mEq/L.

CASE DISCUSSION

This patient suffers from extracellular volume expansion as a result of congestive heart failure. His weight is 14 kg greater than normal, and he has signs of significant fluid accumulation in both his pulmonary interstitium and the interstitial areas of his lower extremities. The inability to ambulate without becoming short of breath (i.e., dyspnea on exertion) and to lie flat (i.e., orthopnea) are important clinical symptoms of fluid accumulation in the pulmonary interstitium. The increase in liver size (i.e., hepatomegaly) and increase in jugular venous distention with hepatic compression (i.e., hepatojugular reflux) are signs of intravascular (i.e., venous) volume expansion.

The urinary sodium excretion in this patient is very low, indicating that he is in a sodium-retaining state. If his GFR was measured, it would be low. If his plasma renin, aldosterone, and angiotensin II concentrations were measured, they would be increased. The renal sympathetic nerve activity also is increased. In addition, the fraction of plasma filtered across the glomerulus is increased; thus, the postglomerular oncotic pressure is increased, promoting increased tubular sodium transport. Therefore, the patient suffers from the stimulation of multiple sodium-retaining reflexes. Inappropriate sodium retention is the primary renal defect in congestive heart failure.

How does cardiac failure result in increased extracellular volume? Congestive heart failure is associated with two primary defects. The cardiac output is diminished, decreasing the effective circulating volume (i.e., the volume of plasma perfusing tissues). The venous pressure is increased. If the right ventricle is impaired, the increased pressure is manifest as right-sided changes, (e.g., jugular distention, hepatomegaly, pedal edema). If the left ventricle is impaired, the increased pressure is manifest as left-sided or pulmonic changes. Increased venous pressure promotes increased Starling's forces favoring the movement of fluid from the capillary space to the interstitium. The decrease in effective circulating volume reflexively increases renin release, angiotensin II formation, and aldosterone activity. Catecholamine levels are also increased in response to a decrease in effective circulating volume. Renin release and renal vascular resistance increase in response to higher plasma catecholamine levels. The increased renal vascular resistance decreases GFR and increases the Starling's forces across the glomerular capillary bed. The increase in filtration fraction results in a higher peritubular capillary Starling's force.

Three factors contribute to a decrease in urinary sodium excretion: increased formation of aldosterone, decreased GFR, and increased peritubular oncotic pressure, which increases tubular sodium reabsorption. On the venous side, increased systemic capillary hydrostatic pressure promotes transudation of fluid into the interstitial space and edema formation. These factors are outlined in Figure 2-11.

Two other clinical disorders commonly result in volume expansion and edema. These are cirrhosis, which is often associated with chronic alcohol inges-

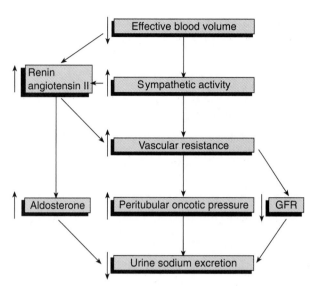

Figure 2-11. Relation between congestive heart failure and decreased urinary sodium excretion. (GFR, glomerular filtration rate.)

tion, and nephrotic syndrome (see Chap. 5). As with congestive heart failure, decreased effective arterial volume is the primary stimulus for renal sodium retention in both disorders. Renin and angiotensin levels are increased. Decreased GFR, increased aldosterone, and increased peritubular oncotic pressure all contribute to decreased urinary sodium excretion. The basis for the decrease in effective circulating volume is different for cirrhosis, nephrotic syndrome, and congestive heart failure. As discussed previously, congestive heart failure results in a fall in effective intraarterial volume as a result of a low cardiac output. Cardiac output is typically normal or elevated in patients with cirrhosis and nephrotic syndrome. In these cases, hypoalbuminemia caused by decreased formation in cirrhosis or urinary protein loss in nephrotic syndrome lowers capillary oncotic pressure and promotes transudation of fluid from the vascular compartments to the interstitial compartments. Two other factors contribute to the fall in effective intraarterial volume in cirrhotics: A high portal pressure is present which causes splanchnic venous pooling, and a low peripheral vascular resistance is present as a result of numerous arteriovenous malformations.

SELECTED READING

Brenner BM, Humes HD. Mechanics of glomerular ultrafiltration. N Engl J Med 1977;297:148.

Briggs JP, Sawaya BE, Schnermann J. Disorders of salt balance. In: Kokko J, Tannen R, eds. Fluids and electrolytes. Philadelphia: WB Saunders, 1990.

Briggs JP, Schnermann J. The tubuloglomerular feedback mechanism: functional and biochemical aspects. Ann Rev Physiol 1986;49:251.

Lippincott's Pathophysiology Series: Renal Pathophysiology, edited by James A. Shayman. J. B. Lippincott Company, Philadelphia © 1995.

Potassium

James A. Shayman

OBJECTIVES

By the end of this chapter the reader should be able to:

- Know the association between K^+ and resting membrane potential.
- Know the factors that influence the distribution of potassium between the intracellular and extracellular fluid.
- Know the major factors that regulate renal potassium excretion (i.e., aldosterone, plasma K^+, distal flow rate, and tubule electronegativity) and the mechanisms by which these factors do so.
- Know the major etiologies of hypokalemia (i.e., decreased intake, cellular redistribution, gastrointestinal loss, and renal loss) and the basis for each cause.
- Know the major causes of hyperkalemia (i.e., increased intake, cellular redistribution, and decreased renal excretion) and the basis for each cause.
- Diagnose simple but clinically significant disorders of potassium balance and know the treatments for these disorders.

Intracellular potassium concentration is high compared with extracellular potassium concentration. This large concentration gradient between intracellular and extracellular potassium is important in the maintenance of the potential difference across cell membranes. The action potentials of muscle and nerve are highly dependent on the transcellular potassium concentration gradient. Disorders of potassium homeostasis are often associated with life-threatening impairments of muscle, cardiac, or neurologic function.

Potassium balance is maintained in two ways. The body regulates potassium concentration internally by regulating the distribution of potassium between intracellular and extracellular compartments. The body regulates potassium concentration externally by controlling renal and extrarenal secretion. Understanding the basic physiology of potassium homeostasis allows the clinician to prevent the development of significant hypokalemia or hyperkalemia or, when these conditions are present, to treat patients appropriately.

PHYSIOLOGY OF POTASSIUM HOMEOSTASIS

The total body potassium content of a typical 70-kg man is approximately 3500 mEq, or 50 mEq/kg body weight; however, only 3% of the potassium is located in exchangeable extracellular compartments (approximately 7.5% of total body potassium is in bone). Thus, the intracellular potassium concentration is about 150 mEq/L, and the extracellular fluid concentration is 4 mEq/L. By definition, an extracellular potassium concentration of less than 3.5 mEq/L is termed *hypokalemia;* an extracellular potassium concentration of more than 5.0 mEq/L is termed *hyperkalemia.*

The standard diet in Western civilization may contain 50 to 100 mEq of potassium per day; in diets in other parts of the world, the amount of potassium ingested may be as high as 500 to 700 mEq per day. Under normal circumstances, the kidney excretes about 90% of the ingested potassium. The remaining potassium is excreted in the stool or, to a lesser degree, in sweat. As renal function falls, the intestinal excretion of potassium rises, and in renal failure, it may be as high as 50% of the total ingested potassium.

PROBLEM 1

Calculate the change in plasma potassium concentration that would occur if a 70-kg person ingested 2 cups of orange juice (20 mEq of potassium) and if none of the potassium was distributed into the intracellular compartment.

ANSWER: The total body water of a 70-kg person is 0.6 L × total body weight, or 42 L. The extracellular fluid is one third of the total body water, or 14 L. Therefore, the change in plasma potassium concentration equals 20 mEq/14 L, or 1.4 mEq/L. If this person's baseline serum potassium concentration was 5.0 mEq/L, rapidly absorbing 20 mEq would cause their serum potassium concentration to rise to 6.4 mEq/L, resulting in significant hyperkalemia. Because significant hyperkalemia does not occur every time a person eats or drinks, additional mechanisms must be present to maintain extracellular potassium concentration.

The extracellular potassium concentration is very tightly regulated. The distribution of intracellular versus extracellular potassium is maintained primarily by Na^+, K^+-ATPase, a transporter found on all cells. This ion exchanger transports 3 sodium ions out of a cell for each 2 potassium ions entering a cell.

The importance of cellular potassium regulation stems in part from the role of potassium in controlling the excitability of cardiac and neuronal tissues. Potassium is of central importance in maintaining the resting membrane potential (E_m). The distribution of any number of cellular ions can contribute to the E_m. However, since the membrane is predominately potassium selective, the cellular and plasma potassium concentrations are the primary determinants of E_m. The membrane potential can be calculated from the Nernst equation:

$$E_m = -61 \, \log([K^+]_c)/([K^+]_e) \qquad [3\text{-}1]$$

PROBLEM 2

Calculate the resting membrane potentials for plasma potassium concentrations of 2.5 mEq/L, 5.0 mEq/L, and 7.5 mEq/L.

ANSWER: Assuming that the intracellular potassium concentration remains at 150 mEq/L, the resting potentials would be −108, −90, and −79 mV, respectively.

Raising the extracellular potassium concentration lowers (i.e., makes less negative) the resting membrane potential, rendering cells more excitable. Lowering the extracellular potassium concentration raises (i.e., makes more negative) the resting membrane potential, rendering cells less excitable, because the resting potential is farther from the threshold potential (Fig. 3-1). The primary clinical manifestations of hypokalemia or hyperkalemia are directly attributable to these effects on membrane potential. Both hypokalemia and hyperkalemia suppress neuromuscular activity and may result in muscle weakness or even paralysis, decreased intestinal motility, and ventricular arrhythmias. The clinical manifestations of potassium disorders are discussed later in this chapter.

To avoid the pathophysiologic consequences of hypokalemia or hyperkalemia, the body requires rapid and efficient mechanisms for maintaining transcellular potassium concentrations and total potassium homeostasis. These requirements are met primarily by the tight regulation of transcellular potassium distribution and renal potassium excretion.

CELLULAR DISTRIBUTION OF POTASSIUM

Factors that affect the cellular distribution of potassium are listed in Table 3-1. The physiologic regulation of transcellular potassium distribution is controlled by several hormones. *Insulin* is one such hormone. Diabetic individuals who are insulin deficient often suffer from hyperkalemia. The mechanism by which insulin regulates potassium uptake has not been definitively determined. In muscle, insulin induces hyperpolarization associated with potassium influx and sodium efflux. This is consistent with the direct activation of Na^+, K^+-ATPase. Insulin may

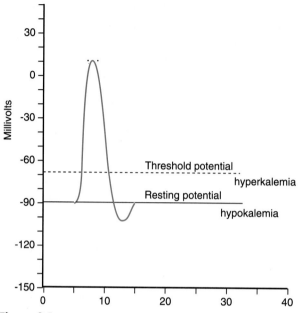

Figure 3-1. Role of potassium in the regulation of the resting membrane potential.

also promote potassium influx through the activation of the Na$^+$, H$^+$ pump. The alkalization of the cell cytosol may also promote potassium uptake. The association between insulin and potassium uptake is bidirectional. Significant changes in plasma potassium concentration affect plasma insulin levels by regulating pancreatic insulin release. Hyperkalemia stimulates and hypokalemia depresses insulin release.

CASE 1

A 45-year-old man is referred to an internist following detection of a blood pressure of 155/95 mm Hg on a routine insurance physical. The internist confirms the presence of hypertension and prescribes a diuretic (hydro-

TABLE 3-1. *FACTORS REGULATING CELLULAR POTASSIUM DISTRIBUTION*

PHYSIOLOGIC	PATHOPHYSIOLOGIC
Insulin	Acid–base status
Catecholamines	Osmolality
Aldosterone	Tissue integrity

chlorothiazide, 25 mg/day). One week later, the patient returns to the internist complaining of polydipsia (i.e., excessive thirst) and polyuria (i.e., frequent urination). What is the basis for the patient's symptoms?

CASE DISCUSSION

On laboratory evaluation, the patient is discovered to have a plasma potassium level of 3.0 mEq/L and a plasma glucose level of 325 mg/dl. The diuretic has caused the hypokalemia by increasing the renal excretion of potassium (discussed later). The hypokalemia has suppressed pancreatic insulin release, resulting in impaired glucose uptake. The hyperglycemia has caused an increase in urine volume due to a limitation on the reabsorption of glucose by the kidney. The increase in urine formation and water loss has stimulated a thirst response in the patient.

Catecholamines cause potassium uptake through activation of β-adrenergic receptors. In peripheral tissues such as muscle this is mediated by the stimulation of β_2-adrenergic receptors and the cAMP-dependent activation of Na^+, K^+-ATPase. The liver and skeletal muscle are the primary sites of potassium uptake. In the heart, β_1 receptors mediate potassium uptake. Although the mechanism for β-adrenergic potassium uptake has not been defined, the benefit of catecholamine-stimulated potassium uptake has an obvious teleological explanation. During trauma or exercise, potassium tends to "leak out" of cells.

An opposing effect of α-adrenergic receptors on promoting hyperkalemia has also been described. This is attributable in part to α-adrenergic–mediated release of potassium from hepatic stores.

Aldosterone may also mediate transcellular potassium distribution by facilitating the movement of potassium into cells. A potential role for aldosterone in regulating potassium distribution is based on studies in adrenalectomized animals. Under these conditions, potassium tolerance is abolished. These studies are inconclusive, however, because the potential effects of catecholamine depletion and alkalosis were not excluded.

A number of pathophysiologic conditions can also affect transcellular potassium concentrations. *Acidosis* promotes potassium egress from cells; *alkalosis* acts oppositely. A rule of thumb is that plasma potassium concentration changes 0.6 mEq/L for each 0.1 pH unit change; however, the basis of the acidosis or alkalosis determines the degree of plasma potassium change. Acidosis caused by excess mineral acids (e.g., ammonium chloride, hydrochloric acid) induce much greater shifts in potassium than do organic acids (e.g., lactic acid, β-hydroxybutyric acid). The shift in potassium from intracellular to extracellular sites because of acute respiratory acidosis is significantly less than that observed as a result of increased mineral acids.

A rapid change in plasma *osmolality* may also induce hyperkalemia. This may occur with an infusion of mannitol or with hyperglycemia accompanying diabetes. Hyperkalemia may be the result of a rapid shift in water from intracellular to extracellular sites, with the movement of potassium occurring as a result of solvent drag. Potassium redistribution also occurs in the setting of *cell injury*. Cell lysis as a result of hemolysis or tissue necrosis may lead to life-threatening hyperkalemia because of the redistribution of potassium into extracellular compartments.

RENAL MECHANISMS FOR POTASSIUM HOMEOSTASIS

Compared with the fraction of sodium excreted, the fraction of potassium that is filtered at the glomerulus and excreted in the final urine is high. The fraction of excreted potassium is usually about 10% to 15% of the filtered potassium. Because the excreted fraction is less than 100% of the filtered fraction, potassium reabsorption must occur. Sometimes, however, the amount of excreted potassium is actually greater than the amount filtered; therefore, a mechanism for the tubular secretion of potassium also must exist.

The tubular handling of potassium by the nephron is outlined in Figure 3-2. Approximately 50% of the filtered potassium is reabsorbed in the proximal convoluted tubule. This reabsorption is primarily diffusion based and is driven across this portion of the nephron by the concentration gradient for potassium. Net potassium secretion occurs in the straight portion of the proximal tubule and the thin descending limb of Henle's loop. The net reabsorption of potassium is the result of the high medullary potassium concentration and a favorable gradient for potassium movement into the nephron. Potassium reabsorption occurs in the thick ascending limb of Henle's loop. This is an extremely efficient process that is driven by both passive and active factors. The positive electrochemical potential of the lumen drives passive potassium reabsorption. Active reabsorption occurs by the Na^+, K^+, Cl^- cotransporter described in Chapter 1. By the end of the thick ascending limb, 90% of the filtered potassium has been reabsorbed.

Tubular transport of potassium through the thick ascending limb is virtually identical in persons on a high-, low-, or normal-potassium diet. Whether a person retains or excretes potassium is determined by the manner in which the potassium is handled in the connecting segment and the cortical collecting duct. Under high-potassium conditions, these structures secrete potassium. Under low-potassium conditions, there is no net potassium secretion. Thus, differences in potassium se-

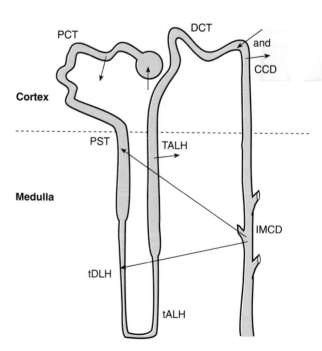

Figure 3-2. Tubular handling of potassium. (CCD, cortical collecting duct; DCT, distal convoluted tubule; IMCD, inner medullary collecting duct; PCT, proximal convoluted tubule; PST, proximal straight tubule; TALH, thick ascending loop of Henle; tALH, thin ascending loop of Henle; tDLH, thin descending loop of Henle.)

cretion are primarily the result of differences in potassium handling by the cortical collecting duct.

The principal cells of the cortical collecting duct are responsible for the net secretion of potassium. The current model for potassium secretion by these cells is shown in Figure 3-3. Energy for potassium secretion is expended in driving Na^+, K^+-ATPase, which transports potassium from the interstitial fluid across the basolateral surface and into the principal cell. This transport creates a high concentration gradient that is favorable for the movement of potassium across potassium channels in the luminal membrane into the tubular lumen. Both the Na^+, K^+-ATPase transporter and the luminal sodium channels are controlled by aldosterone. The luminal membrane has a potential difference that is unfavorable for the movement of potassium. However, the chemical gradient is more favorable to net potassium secretion.

This model of distal tubular potassium secretion is consistent with many of the factors that are known to affect potassium secretion. These factors are listed in Table 3-2.

Ingestion of an excess quantity of potassium will result in an increase in *plasma potassium concentration,* which will increase basolateral potassium transport, resulting in an increase in intracellular potassium concentration. This increase will enhance transport of potassium across the luminal membrane, leading to an increase in tubular potassium secretion. The opposite changes will occur with decreased plasma potassium.

Aldosterone stimulates plasma potassium secretion in two primary ways. This steroid increases the number of basolateral Na^+, K^+-ATPase pumps. Aldosterone also increases the luminal potassium permeability by increasing the number of potassium channels that are in the open position.

Factors affecting the electrochemical gradient for potassium also may profoundly effect potassium secretion. An increased *flow rate* of fluid delivery to the distal convoluted tubule enhances potassium loss. Decreased urinary flow has the opposite effect. Similarly, a change in the transepithelial potential difference will promote or retard the potassium secretory rate. Thus, the delivery of impermeant anions (e.g., sulfate to the distal tubule) may promote potassium loss.

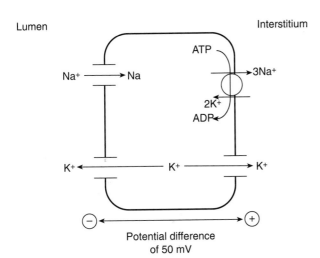

Figure 3-3. Potassium secretion by principal cells of the cortical collecting duct. (ADP, adenosine diphosphate; ATP, adenosine triphosphate.)

TABLE 3-2. *FACTORS REGULATING DISTAL TUBULE POTASSIUM SECRETION*

Plasma potassium concentration
Urinary flow rate
Sodium delivery to the distal tubule
Transepithelial potential difference
Anions
Aldosterone

PROBLEM 3

Diuretics are a class of drugs that promote urinary sodium excretion and thereby result in the loss of extracellular volume. Diuretics act through a variety of mechanisms. Carbonic anhydrase inhibitors block the secretion of hydrogen ions in the proximal tubule and inhibit the reabsorption of bicarbonate and sodium. Loop diuretics block the Na^+, K^+, $2Cl^-$ cotransporter in the thick ascending limb of Henle's loop. Thiazide diuretics inhibit the Na^+, $2Cl^-$ cotransporter in the distal convoluted tubule. Osmotic diuretics inhibit sodium reabsorption as a result of inhibition of the paracellular flux of water. Only the loop diuretics directly block a potassium transporter, yet all of these types of diuretics can cause hypokalemia due to renal potassium loss. What mechanisms account for increased potassium secretion?

ANSWER: Osmotic diuretics and carbonic anhydrase inhibitors inhibit potassium absorption in the proximal tubule. All diuretics increase fluid delivery to the cortical collecting tubule, resulting in enhanced potassium secretion. All forms of diuretics cause sodium depletion, increasing circulating aldosterone, which secondarily stimulates potassium secretion.

EXTRARENAL ROUTES OF POTASSIUM ELIMINATION

Nonrenal routes of potassium loss include the gastrointestinal tract and sweat. Of the typical daily potassium intake (i.e., 50–100 mEq/day), approximately 10% is eliminated in the stool. When renal function is severely compromised, gastrointestinal elimination may account for up to 75% of the total daily intake of potassium. During pathological states (e.g., diarrhea), gastrointestinal potassium loss can be substantial. Under normal conditions, approximately 5 mEq of potassium are lost in the sweat per day. Under more stressful conditions (e.g., physical training, fever) potassium loss can become clinically significant.

HYPOKALEMIA

Hypokalemia refers to a serum or plasma potassium concentration of less than 3.5 mEq/L. This condition can result either from a shift of potassium into the intracellular compartment or from potassium losses of extrarenal or renal origin.

INTRACELLULAR REDISTRIBUTION OF POTASSIUM

CASE 2

A 40-year-old man with a known history of alcohol abuse arrives at the hospital disoriented and hallucinating. His wife notes that he has been on a drinking binge which ended 24 hours before admission. The patient is markedly agitated. Vital signs reveal a regular pulse with a rate of 120 bpm, a blood pressure of 180/100 mm Hg, and a temperature of 102°F. Shortly after admission, the patient suffers a seizure. Laboratory studies show a plasma potassium level of 2.8 mEq/L.

CASE DISCUSSION

This patient is suffering from delirium tremens and seizures as a result of alcohol withdrawal. The abnormalities in his blood pressure, heart rate, and temperature are largely the result of the high levels of circulating catecholamines commonly associated with the cessation of drinking. The patient is also significantly hypokalemic. The basis for his hypokalemia is not the result of loss of potassium from the kidney or from extrarenal sources; rather, his plasma potassium is low because potassium has shifted intracellularly.

Several factors can induce hypokalemia by movement of K^+ into cells. Alkalosis decreases K^+ concentration. An increase in insulin levels caused by hyperglycemia or exogenous insulin administration provokes hypokalemia. Drugs with β_2-agonist properties induce hypokalemia. These drugs include epinephrine and β_2-agonists used to treat asthma and premature labor. As illustrated in Case 2, the endogenous release of catecholamines during acute stressful illnesses such as myocardial infarctions, head injuries, or delirium tremens may lead to hypokalemia. Other intoxicants, including toluene, barium and theophylline, may lead to hypokalemia through cellular shifts. A hereditary disorder, termed hypokalemic periodic paralysis, which is characterized by paralysis and hypokalemia, is the result of intracellular K^+ shifts. Rarely, thyrotoxicosis may result in a similar syndrome.

POTASSIUM DEPLETION SECONDARY TO LOSS

It is useful to subdivide disorders causing K^+ depletion into those due to extrarenal K^+ loss and those due to abnormal renal K^+ wasting. When K^+ depletion is extrarenal in origin, the kidney appropriately conserves K^+. Daily K^+ excretion is less than 20 mEq in this situation.

Extrarenal Causes

K^+ depletion can result from inadequate intake, but the degree of deficiency is usually mild because of appropriate renal K^+ conservation. K^+ depletion can occur in elderly patients on a "tea-and-toast" diet or in women with anorexia nervosa. The latter disorder is often complicated by concomitant K^+ loss as a result of vomiting or diuretic or laxative abuse. Sometimes K^+ depletion results from inadequate intake under conditions in which cell mass is increasing rapidly, for example, during correction of severe anemia. Sweat losses during vigorous training can deplete body K⁺ stores.

The most common cause of extrarenal K⁺ depletion is gastrointestinal loss. Diarrhea is the most frequent cause; the associated metabolic acidosis may provide a diagnostic clue. This problem may occur with laxative abuse. Another less common cause which is not associated with metabolic acidosis is villous adenoma of the rectum.

RENAL CAUSES

For diagnostic purposes, it is useful to subdivide the renal causes of K⁺ depletion based on the associated acid–base status and on the presence of hypertension.

Hypokalemia and Metabolic Acidosis

Hypokalemia is most often associated with metabolic alkalosis or normal acid–base status; therefore, the presence of metabolic acidosis is a useful diagnostic feature. The combination of K⁺ depletion of renal origin and metabolic acidosis is found in renal tubular acidosis (RTA) of either the distal (type I) or proximal (type II) varieties. Acetazolamide and other drugs that inhibit the activity of carbonic anhydrase produce a combination of proximal and distal RTA and thus have a propensity for inducing K⁺ depletion.

Hypokalemic and Metabolic Alkalosis

CASE 3

A 35-year-old woman visits her internist with complaints of headaches that are unresponsive to aspirin. She is hypertensive, with a blood pressure of 170/100 mm Hg. The physical exam is significant for mild hypertensive retinopathy and the absence of an abdominal bruit. Laboratory evaluation reveals the following:

Sodium	135 mEq/L
Potassium	2.5 mEq/L
Chloride	90 mEq/L
Bicarbonate	35 mEq/L
Glucose	90 mg/dl
Blood urea nitrogen	14 mg/dl

Further laboratory evaluation is undertaken. A random plasma renin level is 0.5 ng/ml/hour (normal is 0.9–3.3 ng/ml/hour), and the plasma aldosterone level is 550 ng/L (normal is 10–160 ng/L). An abdominal computed tomographic scan reveals a 3-cm mass in the right adrenal gland.

CASE DISCUSSION

This woman suffers from primary aldosteronism due to an adrenal adenoma. Primary hyperaldosteronism occurring secondary to an adenoma, hyperplasia, or less frequently, a carcinoma, is the classic cause of hypokalemic metabolic alkalosis induced by mineralocorticoid excess. K^+ depletion results from high delivery rates of sodium and fluid to the distal tubule and high levels of aldosterone, leading to net K^+ secretion into the tubular fluid. Other conditions that cause hypertension and hypokalemic alkalosis induced by mineralocorticoid excess include the exogenous ingestion of compounds with mineralocorticoid activity such as licorice (which contains glycyrrhizic acid), carbenoxolone, or fludrocortisone acetate (Florinef), or the topical or intranasal use of corticosteroids with mineralocorticoid activity. In addition, mineralocorticoid-excess syndromes may accompany adrenogenital syndromes caused by either 17α-hydroxylase or 11β-hydroxylase deficiencies. Cushing's syndrome, resulting from the endogenous overproduction or exogenous administration of glucocorticoids, may also produce hypokalemia.

Hypokalemic metabolic alkalosis in the normotensive patient is most often associated with chloride depletion. This syndrome results most frequently from chloride losses from the upper gastrointestinal tract secondary to vomiting or gastric drainage or from renal losses due to diuretic therapy. Other causes include posthypercapneic alkalosis and chloride-losing diarrheal conditions. Chloride depletion results in a mild contraction of the extracellular fluid space and avid renal chloride conservation. In the absence of conditions that interfere with normal renal chloride handling, daily urinary chloride excretion is less than 10 mEq.

Hypokalemia With Variable Acid–Base Status

Other causes of renal K^+ wasting can occur independent of a patient's acid–base status. These conditions include magnesium depletion, which regardless of the cause results in K^+ loss through an undefined mechanism. Antibiotics such as penicillin and its derivatives cause urinary K^+ loss as a result of their anionic properties, which stimulate K^+ secretion by the distal nephron. Gentamicin and other aminoglycoside antibiotics promote renal K^+ wasting by causing direct injury to the tubular epithelium. Hypokalemia may also be seen in association with acute leukemia.

CLINICAL CONSEQUENCES OF HYPOKALEMIA

The functional impact of K^+ depletion results from an increase in the ratio of intracellular to extracellular K^+ concentration. This increased ratio increases the threshold for initiation and impairs the termination of the action potential in excitable tissues.

The most important clinical manifestations of hypokalemia are its effects on the myocardium. Hypokalemia potentiates the effects of cardiac glycosides on myocardial conductivity and can provoke digitalis intoxication. K^+ depletion predisposes the heart to ventricular ectopic rhythms. Ventricular tachycardia and fibrillation occur with increased frequency during myocardial infarction in the presence of hypokalemia. Electrocardiographic evidence of hypokalemia includes prominent U waves (Fig. 3-4).

Neuromuscular manifestations of hypokalemia include malaise, muscular weakness, and cramps. Abnormal bowel motility may result in constipation or ileus. Severe K^+ depletion may provoke life-threatening paralysis involving the respiratory muscles. Rhabdomyolysis may also accompany severe K^+ depletion.

Endocrine complications of K^+ depletion include glucose intolerance sec-

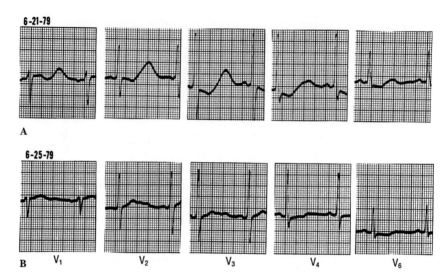

6-21-79

A

6-25-79

B   V₁   V₂   V₃   V₄   V₆

Figure 3-4. The electrocardiogram (ECG) of a hypokalemic patient. **(A)** ECG changes associated with a plasma K⁺ level of 1.3 mEq/L. **(B)** the ECG following normalization of the serum K⁺. (Adapted from Fisch C. Electrocardiography, exercise stress testing, and ambulatory monitoring. In: Kelley WN, ed. Textbook of internal medicine. 2nd ed. Philadelphia: JB Lippincott, 1992:276.)

ondary to defective pancreatic insulin secretion. Additionally there are decreased aldosterone levels. Peripheral vascular resistance is decreased with decreased responsiveness to the vasoconstrictive properties of angiotensin II.

The kidney is affected by K⁺ depletion in several ways. Patients may exhibit polyuria due to impaired concentrating ability in combination with primary polydipsia. Renal vasoconstriction reduces renal blood flow and glomerular filtration rate. Prolonged K⁺ depletion can lead to interstitial nephritis and the development of chronic renal failure. It may also induce the development of renal cysts.

DIAGNOSTIC APPROACH TO HYPOKALEMIA

The underlying cause of the development of hypokalemia is usually apparent from the patient's history and the clinical setting. The history should focus on medications; diet; the existence of vomiting, diarrhea, or other losses of body fluids; and a possible family history of hypokalemia. The physical examination may uncover underlying conditions that can account for the development of hypokalemia. Usually, however, the blood pressure is the most helpful finding, allowing categorization of hypokalemic disorders into diagnostic subsets. The most useful laboratory tests for diagnostic purposes are blood acid–base parameters, urinary K⁺ and chloride values, and occasionally, plasma renin and aldosterone levels. Figures 3-5 and 3-6 provide outlines of approaches to the differential diagnosis of hypokalemic disorders.

TREATMENT OF HYPOKALEMIA

Hypokalemia due to potassium redistribution is usually transient and does not require specific therapy. If serious myocardial sequelae require treatment, the required K⁺ replacement is small because of the lack of an intracellular K⁺ deficit.

Treatment of K⁺ depletion requires decisions about the specific K⁺ salt to be

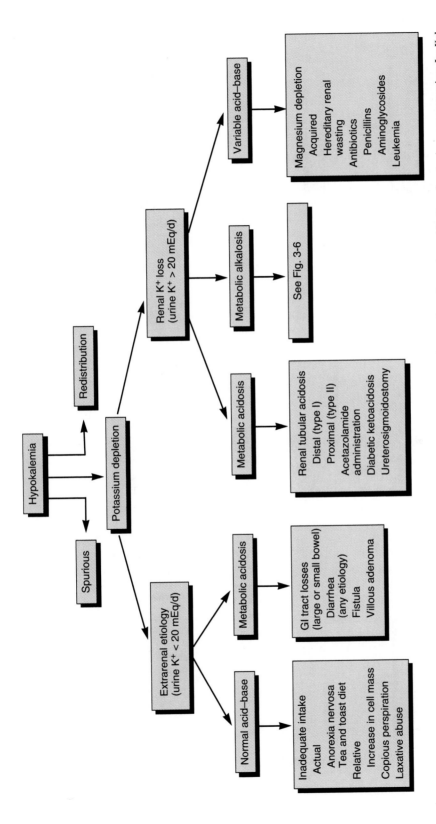

Figure 3-5. Diagnostic approach to hypokalemia. (GI, gastrointestinal.) (From Tannen RL. Approach to the patient with altered potassium concentration. In: Kelley WN, ed. Textbook of internal medicine. 2nd ed. Philadelphia: JB Lippincott, 1992:851.)

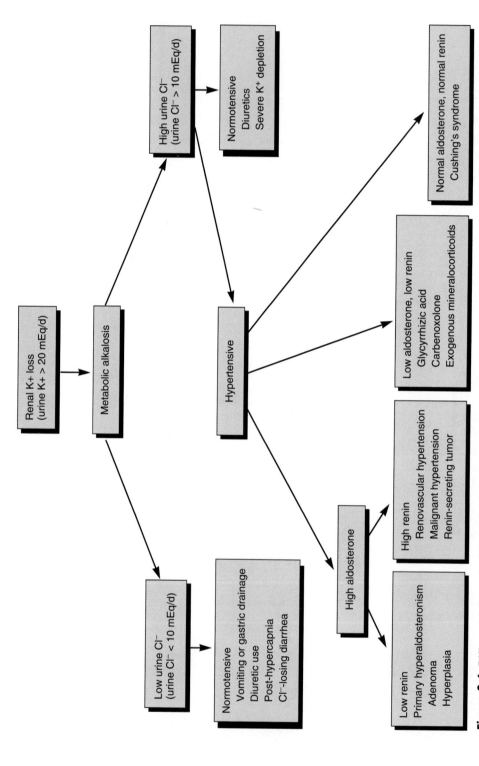

Figure 3-6. Differential diagnosis of hypokalemia associated with metabolic alkalosis and renal potassium wasting. (From Tannen RL. Approach to the patient with altered potassium concentration. In: Kelley WN, ed. Textbook of internal medicine. 2nd ed. Philadelphia: JB Lippincott, 1992:852.)

used and about the route and speed of administration. Assessment of the magnitude of K^+ depletion based on the plasma K^+ concentration may serve as a guide for the amount of K^+ replacement required. The speed of replacement is based on the clinical setting. As a general rule, unless there is a life-threatening emergency, it is prudent to err on the side of slow administration to avoid inducing hyperkalemia. Oral therapy is preferable except when a serious dysrhythmia or paralysis requires rapid correction.

The choice of potassium salt is based on the cause of K^+ depletion. KCl replacement is effective in all circumstances but is absolutely indicated when chloride depletion is the basis for the hypokalemia. In the presence of an associated acidosis, treatment with $KHCO_3$ or the potassium salt of a bicarbonate precursor (e.g., citrate, acetate, gluconate), is a rational choice. Potassium phosphate is a reasonable therapeutic choice when a K^+ and phosphate deficit coexist, such as in diabetic ketoacidosis. In patients receiving diuretic therapy in whom maintenance of a normal plasma K^+ is the goal, potassium-sparing diuretics are often chosen. These include spironolactone, triamterene, and amiloride.

HYPERKALEMIA

Hyperkalemia refers to an elevated serum K^+ value. It may result from a spuriously elevated laboratory value, cellular redistribution from an intracellular to extracellular compartment, or K^+ retention.

SPURIOUS HYPERKALEMIA

Several factors can result in a factitious elevation of serum K^+. These factors include hemolysis of the blood specimen and, rarely, a defect in K^+ permeability of the erythrocyte membrane. Leukocytosis (i.e., white blood cell count >200,000/µl) causes spurious K^+ elevation as a result of K^+ leakage from cells when the cells are preserved at cold temperatures. In contrast, spurious hypokalemia may occur as a result of cellular uptake when the specimen is kept at room temperature. Thrombocytosis (i.e., platelet counts >1,000,000/µl) can elevate K^+ levels as a result of K^+ release during clotting. Excessively tight, prolonged tourniquet application may also elevate K^+ concentration. If a spuriously elevated potassium level is suspected, the determination should be repeated. Confirmation of hyperkalemia by electrocardiographic (ECG) changes should also be performed when the potassium concentration is significantly elevated.

HYPERKALEMIA SECONDARY TO REDISTRIBUTION

The same factors that can cause hypokalemia by shifting K^+ into cells can result in hyperkalemia when their action is opposed. Acidosis, insulin deficiency, and β_2-blocking agents all predispose to hyperkalemia secondary to cellular redistribution. Acidosis is related to hyperkalemia in a complex manner. Only mineral acid or hyperchloremic forms of acidosis result in K^+ shifts, as opposed to organic forms of acidosis, such as lactic acidosis. In addition, the degree of K^+ alteration is greater with metabolic than with respiratory acidosis.

A 25-year-old man with type I (i.e., insulin-dependent) diabetes mellitus comes to the emergency department complaining of having passed out. The patient takes propranolol, a β-adrenergic blocker, for hypertension. The intern draws blood for electrolytes and, assuming that the patient has suffered from a hypoglycemic event, administers an ampule of 50% dextrose in water. Shortly after being given the dextrose, the patient's blood pressure falls, and he suffers a cardiac arrest. A second set of electrolytes are drawn.

Sodium	130 mEq/L	130 mEq/L
Chloride	90 mEq/L	90 mEq/L
Creatinine	1.5 mg/dl	1.5 mg/dl
Potassium	6.5 mEq/L	8.5 mEq/L
Bicarbonate	10 mEq/L	10 mEq/L
Glucose	400 mg/dl	600 mg/dl
Blood urea nitrogen	40 mg/dl	40 mg/dl

CASE DISCUSSION

This is a dramatic example of cardiac arrest as a result of hyperkalemia in a diabetic patient. The basis for the hyperkalemia is redistribution of potassium from intracellular stores. The causes are multifactorial. Insulin-deficient patients with diabetes mellitus are prone to the development of redistribution-induced hyperkalemia. This process is often precipitated by hyperglycemia, because high extracellular osmolality due to hyperglycemia pulls both water and K^+ from the intracellular space. The acidosis (see Chap. 4) caused by high ketoacids causes the egress of potassium from cellular sites. Therapy with β-adrenergic blockers also predisposes toward hyperkalemia due to β-adrenergic receptor blockade.

Other causes of redistribution hyperkalemia include alcohol intoxication or the use of drugs that alter K^+ distribution, such as cardiac glycosides, succinylcholine and other depolarizing muscle relaxants, arginine HCl, and fluoride. K^+ egress from muscle can produce substantial hyperkalemia with acute, maximal, or very prolonged exercise.

HYPERKALEMIA SECONDARY TO K+ RETENTION

K^+ excretion requires a normal number of functioning nephron units, adequate delivery of sodium and fluid to the distal nephron, an intact aldosterone system, and a distal tubular epithelium with an intact K^+ secretory mechanism. Abnormalities in any of these parameters can lead to hyperkalemia.

A 60-year-old man is followed for a 20-year history of essential hypertension. He has moderate renal insufficiency with a baseline creatinine level of

2.5 mg/dl, estimated glomerular filtration rate (GFR) of 20 ml/minute, and a potassium level of 4.0 mEq/L. He has heard that his blood pressure can be better controlled if he decreases his sodium intake. He replaces his table salt with salt substitute. On his next visit to his physician, his creatinine level remains at 2.5 mg/dl, but his potassium is now 5.4 mEq/L.

CASE DISCUSSION

This patient's long-standing hypertension has caused a decreased GFR reflective of a decrease in the number of functioning nephrons. Under these circumstances, the capacity of the kidney to excrete K^+ may be compromised. If K^+ intake is normal, a GFR greater than 5 ml/minute can usually maintain normokalemia. Balance is preserved, because the remaining nephrons adapt their K^+ secretory capacity. Because the kidney is using its adaptive capacity to sustain K^+ balance in the setting of normal intake, hyperkalemia may result when the kidney is presented with an increased K^+ load. This often occurs when the GFR is greater than 5 ml/minute but less than 20 ml/minute. The increased K^+ load may result from exogenous sources such as foods, K^+ replacement therapy, or salt substitutes, or it may result from the endogenous generation of a K^+ load. In the latter case, the K^+ load may arise from tissue trauma, rhabdomyolysis, red cell hemolysis, or bleeding, with subsequent degradation of the red blood cells.

With oliguric or nonoliguric acute renal failure, renal function is so severely impaired that hyperkalemia is a major risk. Every patient who arrives at the hospital with this diagnosis should have an immediate ECG to rule out life-threatening hyperkalemia.

Hyperkalemia may also be observed in the setting of an *adequate GFR*. In this situation, patients have sufficient functioning nephron units for the maintenance of K^+ homeostasis. However, hyperkalemia results from aldosterone deficiency or from a primary defect in K^+ secretion by the distal tubular epithelium.

Aldosterone deficiency, regardless of the underlying cause, predisposes the patient to the development of hyperkalemia. Hypoaldosteronism can result from a primary defect affecting the adrenal gland, such as Addison's disease. Less common causes of hypoaldosteronism include hereditary defects in aldosterone biosynthesis (e.g., adrenogenital syndrome or C21-hydroxylase deficiency). When a low aldosterone level results from a primary defect in adrenal steroid production, plasma renin levels are elevated.

Aldosterone deficiency may also occur in association with chronic renal disease. This type of deficiency is most often associated with tubulointerstitial forms of renal disease and diabetes mellitus. Most of these patients exhibit low renin and aldosterone levels, a syndrome termed hyporeninemic hypoaldosteronism. In addition to hyperkalemia, about one half of these patients exhibit hyperchloremic metabolic acidosis, apparently as a result of hyperkalemia-induced suppression of renal ammonia production and abnormal H^+ secretion as a result of low aldosterone levels. This acidotic syndrome is called type IV RTA.

Several medications can cause hyperkalemia secondary to aldosterone deficiency. Heparin directly impairs adrenal aldosterone biosynthesis; cyclooxygenase inhibitors (e.g., indomethicin) reduce renin release; and angiotensin-converting enzyme inhibitors produce hypoaldosteronism by lowering angiotensin II levels.

Hyperkalemia may also occur in patients with *normal adrenal function*. Several of the diseases that cause hyporeninemic hypoaldosteronism also produce hyperkalemia without a decrease in aldosterone levels. These conditions presumably interfere with K^+ secretion by the distal tubule. These conditions include lupus erythematosus, amyloidosis, obstructive uropathy, sickle cell disease, and postrenal transplantation. The potassium-sparing diuretics all cause tubular hyperkalemia. Spironolactone interferes with the action of aldosterone; amiloride and triamterene inhibit K^+ secretion by an aldosterone-independent mechanism.

CLINICAL CONSEQUENCES OF HYPERKALEMIA

Hyperkalemia alters the function of excitable tissues by decreasing the intracellular-to-extracellular K^+ ratio. The major organ affected is the heart, and severe hyperkalemia can produce cardiac arrest. The ECG manifestations of hyperkalemia parallel the severity and rate of the rise in the K^+ level. Early manifestations are peaking of the T waves. Flattening of the P wave, prolongation of the PR interval, and widening of the QRS complex are seen with more severe hyperkalemia. A final event is a sine wave pattern with cardiac arrest (Fig. 3-7). Hyperkalemia can also produce neurologic symptoms, including tingling, paresthesias, weakness, and flaccid paralysis.

DIAGNOSTIC APPROACH TO HYPERKALEMIA

The assessment of the hyperkalemic patient is outlined in Figure 3-8. The first step in the diagnostic evaluation is to rule out a spurious cause for the hyperkalemia. If the K^+ level is severely elevated, an ECG should be performed promptly.

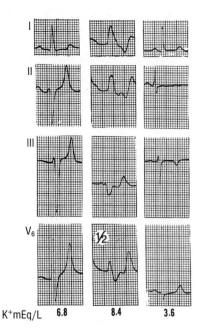

Figure 3-7. The electrocardiogram of a hyperkalemic patient. (From Fisch C. Electrocardiography, exercise stress testing, and ambulatory monitoring. In: Kelley WN, ed. Textbook of internal medicine. 2nd ed. Philadelphia: JB Lippincott, 1992:276.)

K^+mEq/L   6.8   8.4   3.6

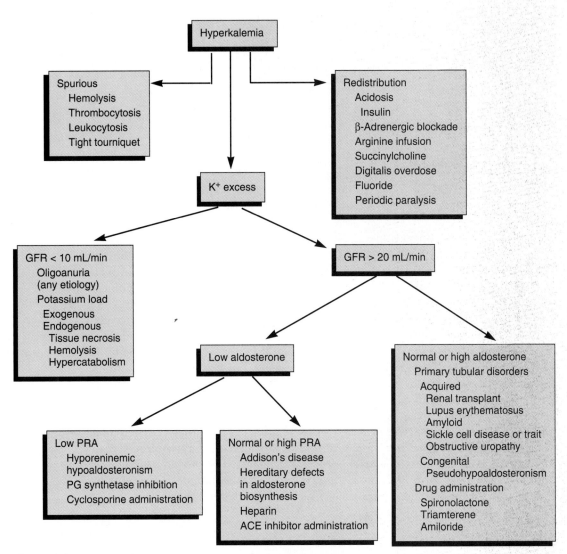

Figure 3-8. Diagnostic approach to hyperkalemia. (ACE, angiotensin-converting enzyme; GFR, glomerular filtration rate; PRA, plasma renin activity.) (From Tannen RL. Approach to the patient with altered potassium concentration. In: Kelley WN, ed. Textbook of internal medicine. 2nd ed. Philadelphia: JB Lippincott, 1992:853.)

The ECG will not only be helpful diagnostically, but it will also dictate the need for the rapid institution of therapy. The next step is to consider the possibility of hyperkalemia due to cellular redistribution by reviewing the clinical situation, determining the acid–base status, and considering drug-induced conditions.

In the presence of oliguria or acute renal failure, the cause of the hyperkalemia is apparent. In more chronic conditions, the measurement of renal function (i.e., plasma creatinine, blood urea nitrogen, and creatinine clearance) is the first step in evaluating hyperkalemia of renal origin. If the GFR is greater than 5 mL/minute, the possibility of either excess K^+ intake or a defect in tubular K^+ secretion must be considered. Hypoaldosteronemic conditions can be determined by measuring of plasma renin and aldosterone levels.

TABLE 3-3. *THERAPY FOR HYPERKALEMIA*	
DRUG	**ONSET OF ACTION**
Calcium gluconate	1–5 min
Sodium bicarbonate	15–30 min
Glucose and insulin	15–30 min
Sodium polystyrene sulfonate	1–2 h

THERAPY

Acute hyperkalemia is a life-threatening abnormality. The vigor of therapy is guided by the plasma K^+ level, the ECG manifestations, and the clinical setting. When the diagnosis is uncertain, it is preferable to err on the side of overtreatment. The therapy for hyperkalemia is outlined in Table 3-3. Calcium antagonizes the effects of hyperkalemia on the heart; bicarbonate and insulin both drive K^+ into the intracellular compartment. β_2-Adrenergic agonists can rapidly induce cellular K^+ uptake, but they are not uniformly effective in patients with renal failure.

Sodium polystyrene sulfonate (Kayexalate) removes K^+ from the body. It works most rapidly when given as a retention enema, but it is also effective when given orally. It sometimes is necessary to use dialysis for K^+ removal. Hemodialysis is much more effective than peritoneal dialysis for this purpose.

Chronic hyperkalemia is most often seen in patients with hyporeninemic hypoaldosteronism. If the K^+ level is less than 5.8 mEq/L, only dietary counseling and avoidance of medications that interfere with K^+ metabolism is required. Treatment options for patients with more significantly elevated K^+ include exogenous mineralocorticoids, loop or thiazide diuretics, and bicarbonate. Occasionally, sodium polystyrene sulfonate (Kayexalate) is recommended for chronic use.

SELECTED READING

DeFronzo R. Hyperkalemia and hyporeninemic hypoaldosteronism. Kidney Int 1980;17:118.

Rose BD. Clinical physiology of acid-base and electrolyte disorders. New York: McGraw-Hill, 1989.

Tannen RL. Potassium disorders. In: Kokko JP, Tannen RL, eds. Fluids and electrolytes. Philadelphia: WB Saunders, 1990.

Lippincott's Pathophysiology Series: Renal Pathophysiology, edited by James A. Shayman. J. B. Lippincott Company, Philadelphia © 1995.

Acids and Bases

Frank C. Brosius

OBJECTIVES

By the end of this chapter the reader should be able to:

- Describe the variables which determine extracellular pH and use the Henderson-Hasselbalch equation (or the nonlogarithmic mass-action equation) to calculate pH or $[H^+]$, pCO_2, and HCO_3^-.
- Identify and understand the function of the major extracellular and intracellular buffering systems.
- Specify the fundamental abnormalities in the four primary acid–base disorders and list several important causes of each disorder.
- Predict the direction and extent of compensation for each of the primary acid–base disorders.
- Use the anion gap as an aid to diagnose the different types of metabolic acidosis.
- Determine when a mixed acid–base disorder is present and identify the associated primary disorders.

The maintenance of a normal acid–base balance and a normal pH is critical for proper enzymatic function and membrane stability. Any significant pH imbalance can result in severe pathology, including respiratory failure, coma, and death. Thus, humans and other animals have developed sophisticated defenses against disruption of normal acid–base balance. In mammals, acute stabilization of acid–base balance after an acid or base load is accomplished by intracellular and extracellular buffers, whereas more chronic regulation of pH is accomplished by two pathways of acid excretion: elimination of carbonic acid by the lungs and elimination of noncarbonic acids by the kidneys. To successfully diagnose different acid–base disorders, it is imperative to have a sound understanding of basic acid–base physiology. Therefore, this chapter begins with a brief review concerning acid–base systems and the control of extracellular pH in the body.

ACID–BASE BALANCE

An acid is any compound that can contribute a proton (H^+) to the extracellular fluid, and a base is any compound that can bind with a proton. The metabolism of carbohydrates, fats, and proteins is the primary source of acid production. The acids formed can be divided into two types, *volatile acids* and *nonvolatile acids*. The major extracellular volatile acid is carbonic acid, which is excreted from the lungs as carbon dioxide. The types of acids formed from the metabolism of these different substrates are shown in Figure 4-1.

The relative daily production rates of volatile versus nonvolatile acids in humans are immensely different; 10,000 to 20,000 mmol of CO_2 are generated from volatile acids daily. In contrast, nonvolatile acid production is approximately 1 mEq/kg body weight/day. Despite this immense acid production, the body maintains the extracellular H^+ ion concentration within a very narrow range (40 ± 5 nM). This is critical because there are many pH-sensitive processes that are vital for normal cellular function. To understand how the body is able to maintain the proton concentration within such a narrow range, it is important to review the concept of buffering.

Any acid can be considered to be in an equilibrium between its dissociated and nondissociated forms.

$$H^+ + A^- \leftrightarrow HA \qquad [4\text{-}1]$$

The ratio of the concentrations of the free proton, free anion, and associated proton–anion pair can be expressed as an association constant (K_a).

$$K_a = [H^+]\,[A^-]\,/\,[HA] \qquad [4\text{-}2]$$

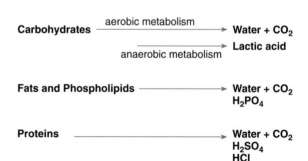

Figure 4-1. Acids formed by substrate metabolism.

Solving for [H⁺]

$$[H^+] = K_a ([HA]/[A^-])$$

By taking the negative logarithm of each side:

$$-\log[H^+] = -\log K_a -\log [HA]/[A^-]$$ [4-3]

pH is the same as $-\log[H^+]$, and pK_a can be used as a notation for $-\log K_a$. By rearranging the signs, the following equation is derived.

$$-\log[H^+] = -\log K_a +\log[A^-]/[HA]$$

This is the *Henderson-Hasselbalch equation*. This equation allows the pH of an acid–base system to be calculated from the molar ratio of the acid and base and pK_a, or alternatively, to determine the molar ratio of the acid and base when the pH and pK_a are known.

A buffer is any system that tends to resist a change in pH when either acid or base is added. Several potential buffers are present both intracellularly and extracellularly. These include proteins, phosphate, and bicarbonate. The relative contributions of these buffers in a closed system can be determined by comparing their titration curves following the addition of acid (Fig. 4-2). The midpoint of the titration curve is equal to the pK_a of the acid.

By this type of analysis, the pK_as for proteins, phosphate, and bicarbonate buffers are the following:

$$H\text{-protein} \leftrightarrow H^+ + \text{protein}^-, pK_a = 7.4$$

$$H_2PO_4 \leftrightarrow H^+ + HPO_4^{-2}, pK_a = 6.8$$

$$H^+ + HCO_3^- \leftrightarrow H_2CO_3 \leftrightarrow H_2O + CO_2, pK_a = 6.1$$

Although not measured clinically, intracellular buffers play an important role in minimizing the effect of acid or base loads on intracellular and extracellular pH. The major intracellular buffers are proteins and inorganic and organic phos-

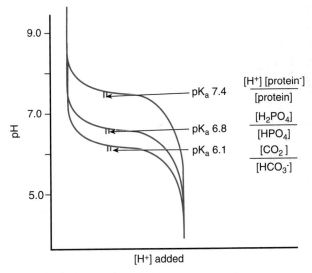

Figure 4-2. The association between pK_a and different physiologic buffers.

phates. Intracellular buffers are responsible for buffering more than 50% of a non-carbonic acid load and virtually all of a carbonic acid load.

In principle, proteins should provide the greatest extracellular buffering capacity, because their average pK_a is close to that of the pH of plasma (7.4). However, bicarbonate provides the major buffer in the body, despite the fact that its pK_a is more than 1 unit less than the pH of plasma. The CO_2–bicarbonate system is the major extracellular buffer system for two reasons: the bicarbonate concentration is very high in plasma (24 mmolar), and the bicarbonate system is not a closed one. CO_2 formed from the dissociation of carbonic acid is rapidly removed by respiration. In other words, *CO_2 is in dynamic equilibrium with H^+.*

The concentration of H_2CO_3, H^+, and HCO_3^- can be substituted as a measure of the major buffer in the plasma.

$$pH = pK + \log[HCO_3^-]/[H_2CO_3] \hspace{2cm} [4\text{-}4]$$

The concentration of CO_2 dissolved in blood is more than 800 times greater than the carbonic acid (H_2CO_3) concentration. Therefore, H^+ is normally related to the partial pressure of CO_2 directly by the following substitution.

$$pH = pK + \log[HCO_3^-]/\alpha\, pCO_2$$

where α represents the solubility constant for CO_2 in water (0.03).

This equation can be rewritten as a simple mass-action equation:

$$[H^+] = 24(pCO_2)/[HCO_3^-]$$

This is a clinically useful equation, because $[HCO_3^-]$ and pCO_2 are routinely measured. The relation between $[H^+]$ and pH over a physiologically relevant range is shown in Table 4-1.

As this table demonstrates, a pH decrease of only 0.3 (e.g., from 7.4 to 7.1) corresponds to a doubling of the H^+ concentration.

PROBLEM 1

If the association of CO_2 and H_2O results in the formation of one molecule of HCO_3^- and H^+, then why does a doubling in plasma pCO_2 (40–80 mm Hg) result in a fall in plasma pH?

ANSWER: Increasing pCO_2 to 80 mm Hg, increases $[H^+]$ from 40 to 80 nmoles/L. The normal $[HCO_3^-]$ is 24 mmol/L. Therefore, under normal conditions, $[H^+] = 24(40\ \text{mm Hg})/(24\ \text{mEq/L}) = 40\ \text{nM}$; but under conditions of pCO_2 retention, $[H^+] = 24(80\ \text{mm Hg})/(24.00004\ \text{mEq/L}) = 80\ \text{nM}$. In other words, the concentration of HCO_3^- in the plasma is much greater than the concentration of H^+. Thus, a change in pCO_2 results in a proportionately greater change in $[H^+]$ compared with $[HCO_3^-]$.

TABLE 4-1.   *RELATION BETWEEN PH AND H⁺ CONCENTRATION*

pH	6.8	6.9	7.0	7.1	7.2	7.3	7.4	7.5	7.6	7.7	7.8
$[H^+]$ (nM)	160	125	100	80	63	50	40	32	26	20	16

To understand the importance of the intracellular and extracellular buffering systems in protecting the body from major changes in H$^+$ concentration, it is helpful to consider the following hypothetical case of how a person would handle an acute acid load.

PROBLEM 2

A 70-kg man is given a 35-mmole infusion of hydrochloric acid. Initially, the H$^+$ ions are constrained to the vascular compartment. However, in 10 to 15 minutes, the H$^+$ equilibrates with the entire extracellular space. Within 2 to 3 hours, the H$^+$ equilibrates with the intracellular compartment. Initially the entire 35 mmoles of H$^+$ is buffered by the HCO$_3^-$ in the blood. Because the plasma volume is approximately 3 Ls (see Chap. 2), the plasma HCO$_3^-$ concentration will fall by 35 mmoles/3 L, or 11.7 mmolar, or from 24 to 12.3 mmolar.

If within minutes the acid is distributed throughout the entire extracellular space (14 L), the HCO$_3^-$ concentration would be 24 mmolar − 35 mmole/14 L = 21.5 mmolar. Within a few hours, more than 50% of the acid is distributed into the intracellular compartment, so that only 15 mmoles of the H$^+$ would be buffered against extracellular HCO$_3^-$. Therefore, the final HCO$_3^-$ concentration would be 24 mmolar − 15 mmoles/14 L = 23 mmolar.

Use the Henderson-Hasselbalch equation to calculate this hypothetical patient's pH, assuming that there is no change in pCO$_2$ (40 mm Hg).

ANSWER

$$[H^+] = 24(pCO_2)/[HCO_3^-]$$

Substituting the derived values given above for HCO$_3^-$ concentrations provide the values shown in Table 4-2.

These calculations are hypothetical, because the normal individual would compensate to an acid challenge by increasing ventilation and reducing pCO$_2$.

RESPIRATORY MECHANISMS OF ACID–BASE BALANCE

As stated previously, the normal individual produces approximately 15,000 mEq of carbonic acid daily. This carbonic acid load may increase up to 20-fold during extreme exercise. Despite this impressive amount of acid production, the body maintains its H$^+$ concentration within very narrow limits (35–45 nmolar; pH

TABLE 4-2.

	HCO$_3^-$ (mEq/L)	H$^+$ (nM)	pH
Immediate	12.3	78	7.1
Minutes later	21.5	44.7	7.35
Hours later	23	41.7	7.38

7.35–7.45). The major site of finely regulated CO_2 excretion is the lungs, which are able to maintain the pCO_2 at the appropriate level despite major excursions in carbonic acid production.

The high solubility and diffusibility of CO_2 in water make it a particularly useful vehicle for the delivery of acid from tissues to blood. The CO_2-carrying capacity of the red blood cell is aided by two phenomena: carbonic anhydrase in the red cell converts much of the CO_2 to HCO_3^-, which is rapidly transported out of the red cell into the plasma; and CO_2 forms a carbamino compound with hemoglobin. The formation of the carbamino compound is greater with reduced hemoglobin and less with oxyhemoglobin; thus, binding is enhanced in peripheral tissues, where oxygen levels are low. In the lungs, both processes are reversed, and CO_2 is rapidly released.

The control of CO_2 excretion is accomplished by changes in the rate and volume of ventilation in the lung (i.e., minute ventilation). An increase in alveolar minute ventilation results in a decrease in arterial pCO_2; a decrease in alveolar minute ventilation results in an increase in arterial pCO_2. The afferent signals for changing minute ventilation emanate from respiratory chemoreceptors that regulate the central drive for respiration. There are two types of chemoreceptors: CO_2 receptors located in the medulla oblongata, aortic body, and carotid bodies; and pH receptors located in the carotid body. The lungs are the first line of defense in the maintenance of acid–base homeostasis, because they provide a mechanism for the almost immediate regulation of acid excretion.

RENAL MECHANISMS OF ACID–BASE BALANCE

Although the formation of nonvolatile acids is quantitatively small compared to the formation of volatile acids, it is the function of the kidney to excrete the 50 to 100 mEq/day of nonvolatile acids formed from the metabolism of protein and other substrates. The excretion of nonvolatile acid occurs in the collecting tubule, where protons are secreted and are buffered by phosphate and sulfate (i.e., titratable acids) and by ammonia. However, before net acid excretion can occur, the kidneys must reabsorb the HCO_3^- which is filtered at the glomerulus.

PROBLEM 3

Calculate the daily filtered load of HCO_3^-. Assume an average plasma HCO_3^- of 24 mEq/L and glomerular filtration rate (GFR) of 120 ml/minute.

ANSWER

Filtered load HCO_3^- = (24 mEq/L) (0.120 L/minute) (1440 minutes/day)
$$= 4147 \text{ mEq/day}$$

The efficiency of the kidney in reclaiming HCO_3^- is very high. An average person may excrete less than 5 mEq of HCO_3^- per day. Table 4-3 compares the amount of filtered HCO_3^- and forms of daily acid excretion.

The most important site of HCO_3^- reclamation is the proximal tubule, where 90% of reabsorption occurs. However, this does not occur by direct transport of HCO_3^- across the luminal membrane. Rather, H^+ from carbonic acid formed from water and CO_2 by carbonic anhydrase, is actively transported across the luminal

TABLE 4-3. *THE RELATION BETWEEN FILTERED BICARBONATE AND NET ACID EXCRETION*

ACID OR BASE	mEq/DAY
Filtered HCO_3^-	4150
Tubular reabsorption of HCO_3^-	4145
Urinary HCO_3^- excretion	5
Urinary titratable acid excretion	55
Urinary ammonium excretion	30
Net acid excretion	80

membrane by a Na^+, H^+ exchanger. The HCO_3^- is then transported across the basolateral surface. The secreted H^+ rapidly combines with the filtered HCO_3^-, forming carbonic acid (H_2CO_3). Carbonic acid is converted to water and carbon dioxide by carbonic anhydrase (CA) on the luminal side of the proximal tubule brush border. The CO_2 diffuses back into the proximal tubule cells, where it combines with H_2O to form carbonic acid to complete the cycle (Fig. 4-3).

The daily noncarbonic acid load is secreted by the intercalated cells of the cortical and outer medullary collecting ducts. The secretion of H^+ into the tubular lumen is accomplished by a H^+-ATPase, whereas HCO_3^- reabsorption across the basolateral surface is mediated by a chloride, HCO_3^- exchanger (Fig. 4-4).

The amount of acid excreted is critically dependent on the presence of urinary buffers. The maximum pH of the collecting tubule luminal fluid is 4.0 (H^+ = 0.1 mEq/L). Therefore, only 0.1% to 0.2% of the daily load of 50 to 100 mEq of acid can be excreted as nonbuffered H^+. The remainder of urinary H^+ must be excreted in buffered form, usually as phosphates or ammonium. The concentration of ammonium is primarily regulated by the kidney and varies depending on total

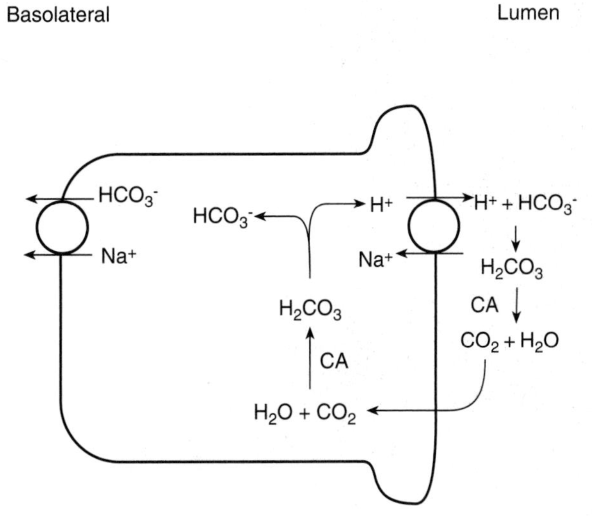

Figure 4-3. Proximal tubule cell bicarbonate reabsorption. (CA, carbonic anhydrase.)

Basolateral   Lumen

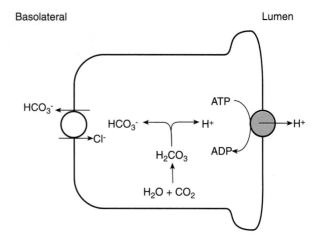

Figure 4-4. Collecting tubule α-intercalated cell H^+ secretion. (ADP, adenosine diphosphate; ATP, adenosine triphosphate.)

body acid–base balance. Thus, daily acid secretion is largely dependent on the amount of ammonium excreted (Fig. 4-5).

Several factors regulate acid secretion by both the proximal and collecting tubules. (Table 4-4). Some factors are important because they affect substrate dependence (e.g., pCO_2). Other factors are important because they affect the electrochemical gradient regulating proton transport or the amount of buffer available. For example, aldosterone promotes H^+ secretion by two mechanisms: the mineralocorticoid stimulates Na^+ reabsorption and increases the negative voltage of the lumen, which is favorable for H^+ secretion; and aldosterone directly stimulates the H^+-ATPase.

In contrast with the rapid pulmonary response to changes in acid–base status,

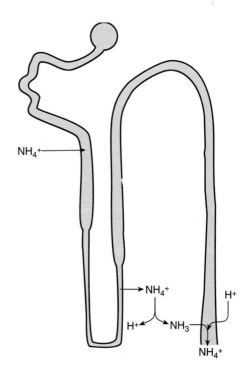

Figure 4-5. NH_3, NH_4^+ handling by the kidney. NH_4^+ is produced and secreted by the proximal tubule cells. It is then reabsorbed by the ascending loop of Henle and concentrated in the renal medulla. A small amount of NH_4^+ dissociates into NH_3 and H^+. The H^+ is reabsorbed, but the NH_3 can diffuse into the collecting tubule, where it can buffer the H^+ ions secreted by the intercalated cells.

TABLE 4-4. *REGULATORS OF H^+ AND HCO_3^- TRANSPORT*	
PROXIMAL TUBULE	**COLLECTING TUBULE**
pCO_2	pH gradient
Filtered HCO_3^- load	Electrical potential difference
Carbonic anhydrase function	pCO_2
Parathyroid hormone	Aldosterone
Serum K^+ and PO_4^-	NH_4^+ excretion

the renal response is slow. The stimulation of tubular H^+ secretion by changes in pCO_2 begins to occur after several minutes. However, the stimulation of distal tubular H^+ secretion by aldosterone occurs over the course of hours, and other factors that modulate renal H^+ excretion may take up to 2 to 3 days to be fully expressed. Compensatory renal adaptations to acidosis or alkalosis take place, but these changes are chronic in nature.

PRIMARY ACID–BASE DISORDERS

Primary or simple acid–base disorders are conditions in which only one acid–base abnormality is present. A *primary respiratory acidosis* is caused by an increase in pCO_2, and a *primary respiratory alkalosis* is caused by a decrease in pCO_2. *Metabolic acidosis* is caused by a decrease in HCO_3^- through buffering of H^+ from noncarbonic acids, and *metabolic alkalosis* is caused by an increase in HCO_3^-.

RESPIRATORY ACIDOSIS

Hypoventilation results in *hypercapnia* (i.e., increased pCO_2) and an increase in the H^+ concentration. Multiple processes may result in hypoventilation; these may be operationally divided into acute and chronic processes (Table 4-5).

The observed response to a respiratory acidosis depends on whether an assessment is made early following the development of an acute respiratory acidosis or during a well-established chronic respiratory acidosis. Following an acute respiratory acidosis, plasma HCO_3^- increases modestly to limit the change in pH. The renal compensatory responses to an acid load are slow; therefore the increase in plasma HCO_3^- is not the result of renal mechanisms but is the result of cellular and extracellular buffering. The increase in H^+ concentration is partially buffered by plasma proteins; however, this accounts for no more than 10% of the acute increase in HCO_3^-. The major change in HCO_3^- occurs as a result of buffering by hemoglobin and other tissue buffers. Chloride is exchanged for intracellular HCO_3^-; thus the change in plasma HCO_3^- is known as the *chloride shift*. In acute respiratory acidosis, $[HCO_3^-]$ increases by 0.1 mEq/L for each 1 mm Hg increase in arterial pCO_2.

If the respiratory acidosis is chronic, the increase in plasma HCO_3^- is amplified by increased HCO_3^- retention by the kidney. Urinary ammonium excretion

TABLE 4-5.	*CAUSES OF RESPIRATORY ACIDOSIS*
Acute respiratory acidosis	Acute airway obstruction
	Central nervous system depression (e.g., drug intoxication)
	Cardiac arrest
	Neuromuscular defects (e.g., Guillain-Barré syndrome)
	Chest wall trauma or pneumothorax
	Acute parenchymal lung disorders (e.g., severe pneumonias, respiratory distress, syndrome, pulmonary edema
Chronic respiratory acidosis	Chronic obstructive pulmonary disease
	Respiratory center depression
	Neuromuscular defects (e.g., multiple sclerosis, muscular dystrophy, amyotrophic lateral sclerosis)
	Restrictive defects (e.g., kyphoscoliosis)

increases, and tubular reabsorption of HCO_3^- is enhanced. Following chronic compensation, HCO_3^- increases by 0.3 mEq/L for each 1 mm Hg increase in arterial pCO_2.

RESPIRATORY ALKALOSIS

Excessive ventilation relative to CO_2 production results in primary respiratory alkalosis, or *hypocapnia*. Primary respiratory alkalosis constitutes one of the most common acid–base disorders. Hyperventilation may be the result of any of several processes (Table 4-6). Although many of these processes are benign, many are life-threatening and when present indicate a poor prognosis for the patient.

By mechanisms comparable to primary respiratory acidosis, the adaptation to acute hypercapnia is associated with an immediate fall in plasma HCO_3^-. HCO_3^- decreases as a result of nonrenal mechanisms, primarily by titration with intracellu-

TABLE 4-6.	*CAUSES OF RESPIRATORY ALKALOSIS*

Hypoxemia
Central nervous system diseases (e.g., stroke, tumor, infection)
Drugs (e.g., salicylates, xanthines, adrenergic agonists)
Pregnancy
Hepatic insufficiency
Gram-negative sepsis
Anxiety
Pulmonary disease (e.g., pneumonia, asthma, pulmonary embolus)
Mechanical overventilation

lar nonbicarbonate buffers. The plasma HCO_3^- falls by 0.2 mEq/L for each mm Hg decrement in pCO_2. Chronic adaptation occurs at the level of the kidney. H^+ secretion is decreased and is manifest by a fall in ammonium secretion and suppression of HCO_3^- reabsorption. This adaptation occurs over 2 to 3 days. On average, the plasma HCO_3^- falls by 0.4 to 0.5 mEq/L for each mm Hg decrement in pCO_2.

CASE 1

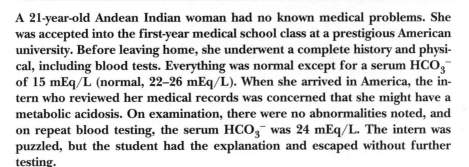

A 21-year-old Andean Indian woman had no known medical problems. She was accepted into the first-year medical school class at a prestigious American university. Before leaving home, she underwent a complete history and physical, including blood tests. Everything was normal except for a serum HCO_3^- of 15 mEq/L (normal, 22–26 mEq/L). When she arrived in America, the intern who reviewed her medical records was concerned that she might have a metabolic acidosis. On examination, there were no abnormalities noted, and on repeat blood testing, the serum HCO_3^- was 24 mEq/L. The intern was puzzled, but the student had the explanation and escaped without further testing.

CASE DISCUSSION

This case illustrates several important concepts in the diagnostic approach to a patient with a potential acid–base disorder. Contrary to the expectation of the intern, the Andean student did not have metabolic acidosis, but instead had a chronic respiratory alkalosis. The mass action equation $H^+ = 24 \times pCO_2/HCO_3^-$ illustrates that the H^+ is dependent on *both* pCO_2 and HCO_3^-. Therefore, it is impossible to reliably make the diagnosis of an acid–base disorder when only one of those critical laboratory values is known. In other words, a low HCO_3^- does not necessarily mean that the H^+ is increased. If the pCO_2 is also decreased, so that the ratio of pCO_2 to HCO_3^- is low, the H^+ will also be low. This is exactly what happened in the case of the Andean student.

For people living at extreme elevations, hypoxia caused by low ambient atmospheric oxygen levels causes a chronic increase in ventilation and decrease in pCO_2. As noted previously, renal mechanisms compensate for the low pCO_2 by decreasing renal ammonium excretion and bicarbonate reabsorption, thereby decreasing the $[HCO_3^-]$. This normal compensatory change was the only "abnormality" found in the medical student's initial laboratory evaluation. Had a complete (and unnecessary) evaluation been conducted, including an arterial blood gas, the decreased pCO_2 and decreased H^+ would have been detected. The lack of any metabolic abnormality was proven when the student descended to an elevation with normal atmospheric oxygen levels. Without the need for increased ventilation, the pCO_2 rapidly rose to normal levels, and somewhat more slowly, the HCO_3^- level also rose to normal levels, as documented by the second set of laboratory values.

METABOLIC ACIDOSIS

Metabolic acidoses comprise a large proportion of the critical acid–base disorders encountered in clinical situations. In most cases, it is imperative to quickly diagnose the cause of the metabolic acidosis to initiate appropriate intervention. Metabolic acidoses generally fall into two groups. The first group is comprised of those conditions in which the noncarbonic acid being added is HCl. Addition of HCl causes a decrease in the HCO_3^- concentration, which is matched by an increase in Cl^- concentration ($HCl + HCO_3^- \rightarrow H_2CO_3 + Cl^-$). Therefore, this type of metabolic acidosis is sometimes referred to as *hyperchloremic* metabolic acidosis (Table 4-7).

Many of the causes of hyperchloremic metabolic acidosis are intuitively obvious, such as the infusion of an acid containing chloride as its anion. Bicarbonate loss occurs from the gastrointestinal tract or is evident during recovery from chronic respiratory alkalosis, when cessation of the renal compensatory response takes several days to occur, and therefore the $[HCO_3^-]$ remains low despite normal pCO_2. Such a phenomenon would have occurred in the case of the Andean medical student for the first day or two after moving to sea level. Types I and II renal tubular acidoses are conditions in which there is a defect in bicarbonate reclamation or acid secretion in the distal or proximal nephron, respectively.

The second group of metabolic acidoses is comprised of those conditions in which the acid is not HCl (e.g., lactic acid in lactic acidosis). When non-HCl acids accumulate, the HCO_3^- concentration is reduced without an increase in Cl^- ($HA + HCO_3^- \rightarrow H_2CO_3 + A^-$). This type of acidosis is usually termed a *high anion gap acidosis*. The anion gap is a somewhat artificial but extremely helpful laboratory value, and is calculated as follows:

$$\text{anion gap} = [Na^+] - ([Cl^-] + [HCO_3^-]).$$ [4-5]

The difference between the concentration of sodium and the sum of chloride and bicarbonate concentrations is the gap between the usually measured cations and the usually measured anions. Potassium is usually ignored because its concentra-

---

TABLE 4-7.   *CAUSES OF HYPERCHLOREMIC METABOLIC ACIDOSES*

Exogenous acid load	Hydrochloric acid
	Arginine chloride
	Ammonium chloride
	Hyperalimentation solutions
Bicarbonate loss or dilution	Gastrointestinal losses (e.g., severe diarrhea, pancreatic or small bowel fistula, ureterosigmoidostomy)
	Recovery from respiratory alkalosis
	Sudden volume expansion
Decreased renal acid secretion	Proximal renal tubular acidosis (RTA type II)
	Distal RTA (type I)
	Hypoaldosteronism

tion proportionately varies so little. Because electroneutrality must be preserved, the gap reflects the concentration of unmeasured anions (A^-, in Equation 4-5). The usual value of the anion gap is 12 ± 4 mEq/L. In a hyperchloremic acidosis, HCl accumulates, and every decrease in HCO_3^- concentration is matched by an increase in Cl^- concentration; therefore, the anion gap remains normal. However, when another acid accumulates, the HCO_3^- is replaced by another anion (A^-) which is not conventionally measured (e.g., lactate, ketoacids, sulfates). Therefore, the sum of $[Cl^-] + [HCO_3^-]$ is decreased, and the gap increases.

Only a limited number of conditions produce a metabolic acidosis with an elevated anion gap (Table 4-8). Therefore, determining the anion gap in a patient with metabolic acidosis often helps in the diagnostic search for the cause of the disorder.

The response of the body to a fall in HCO_3^- is directed at reducing the degree of acidemia. Initially, the additional H^+ are buffered by HCO_3^- and intracellular buffers, such as hemoglobin. The fall in pH also stimulates the central chemoreceptors to increase minute ventilation. The decrease in pCO_2 that occurs in response to the fall in pH occurs rapidly, and therefore is essentially the same whether the metabolic acidosis is acute or chronic. The decrease in pCO_2 is expressed by the following equation:

$$\text{decrease in } pCO_2 = (1.2)(\text{decrease in } [HCO_3^-])$$

When the fall in pCO_2 deviates from this expected change, then another acid–base disturbance is present.

As discussed in Chapter 3, an increase in plasma K^+ concentration is also observed in the setting of acute metabolic acidosis. This change is the result of the shift of intracellular potassium to the extracellular compartment. However, the association between acidosis and hyperkalemia is often difficult to predict. For example, mineral acid infusions with HCl are associated with hyperkalemia, whereas organic acid infusions with lactate are not. In addition, other factors such as glucose, insulin, and catecholamines may alter plasma K^+ concentrations.

METABOLIC ALKALOSIS

Metabolic alkalosis is characterized by increased HCO_3^- and decreased H^+ and Cl^- in the extracellular fluid. The basis for these disorders is either the loss of H^+ or exposure to an exogenous load of HCO_3^- (Table 4-9).

TABLE 4-8. *CONDITIONS ASSOCIATED WITH AN ANION GAP ACIDOSIS*

Ketoacidosis (e.g., diabetes mellitus, starvation, ethanol ingestion)

Uremia

Methanol, toluene, and ethylene glycol intoxication

Lactic acidosis (e.g., hypoxia, poor tissue perfusion, shock, carbon monoxide poisoning, multiple drug ingestions, glucose-6-phosphatase deficiency)

Paraldehyde ingestion

TABLE 4-9. *CAUSES OF METABOLIC ALKALOSIS*	
Increased bicarbonate load	Sodium bicarbonate therapy, seen after treatment of high anion gap metabolic acidoses with HCO_3^-; the accumulated acidic anions (e.g., lactate) are metabolized to HCO_3^- or are excreted, leaving the extra HCO_3^- behind
	Milk–alkali syndrome
	Gastrointestinal losses (e.g., severe vomiting, villous adenoma)
Loss of H^+ ions	
Chloride-responsive alkalosis (urine Cl^- < 10 mEq/L)	Diuretics
	Recovery from respiratory acidosis, ketoacidosis, or lactic acidosis
	Unreabsorbed anion (e.g., carbenicillin, ticarcillin)
Chloride-unresponsive alkalosis (urine Cl^- > 20 mEq/L)	Increased renin states (e.g., accelerated hypertension, renovascular hypertension)
	Primary hyperaldosteronism
	Cushing's syndrome, including exogenous steroid therapy
	Congenital adrenal hyperplasia
	Bartter's syndrome

Causes of metabolic alkalosis as a result of H^+ loss can be categorized based on whether they are accompanied (and caused in part) by depletion of Cl^- from the extracellular space. The urinary Cl^- concentration invariably is low in patients with these disorders. These chloride-responsive metabolic alkaloses improve when patients receive NaCl. The chloride-unresponsive alkaloses do not respond to such treatment, have high urinary Cl^- concentrations, and generally are caused by abnormalities in the renin–angiotensin II–aldosterone system.

SUMMARY OF THE COMPENSATORY CHANGES IN RESPONSE TO PRIMARY RESPIRATORY AND METABOLIC ACID–BASE DISTURBANCES

To maintain the stability of intracellular and extracellular pH, the body compensates for primary acid–base disorders by returning the ratio of extracellular pCO_2 to HCO_3^- to near normal. For example, if the primary acid–base disorder is a metabolic acidosis, the HCO_3^- concentration falls, causing an increase in the ratio of pCO_2 to HCO_3^- and an increase in H^+ concentration. The body compensates for this change by augmenting ventilation, which decreases the pCO_2, thereby returning the pCO_2-to-HCO_3^- ratio to near normal. If the primary disorder is a respiratory acidosis, the pCO_2 is increased, thus increasing the pCO_2-to-HCO_3^- ratio. Intracellular buffering and eventually renal mechanisms compensate by increasing

$[HCO_3^-]$ in the extracellular space, and returning the pCO_2-to-HCO_3^- ratio to near normal.

It is important to recognize that such *compensatory changes do not completely correct the abnormal pH*. Patients with primary metabolic acidosis and primary respiratory acidoses have persistently decreased pH or increased H^+, and patients with primary metabolic or respiratory alkaloses have persistently increased pH or decreased H^+. Table 4-10 depicts the predicted magnitude of the compensatory responses for the four primary acid–base disorders.

PROBLEM 4

A 45-year-old woman had persistent diarrhea for 2 days. On examination, she was tachypneic, with a respiratory rate of 22 breaths/minute. Her blood gases and other laboratory values were as follows: arterial pH, 7.20; pCO_2, 19 mm Hg; HCO_3^-, 7 mEq/L; Na^+, 140 mEq/L; K^+, 4.7 mEq/L; Cl^-, 122 mEq/L. What is her acid–base disorder, and what is the likely cause? What is her anion gap? What is the cause of her tachypnea? How should she be treated?

ANSWERS: Diarrhea causes significant HCO_3^- losses from the gastrointestinal tract, equivalent to the addition of HCl. The anion gap is 140 mEq/L – (122 mEq/L + 7 mEq/L) = 11 mEq/L, which is normal. Therefore, this patient has a hyperchloremic metabolic acidosis. The tachypnea reflects respiratory compensation for a metabolic acidosis and is responsible for the decreased pCO_2. The predicted compensation is a decrease in pCO_2 of 1.2 × (D HCO_3^-) = 20.4, which is essentially equal to that observed in this patient. Thus, the decrease in pCO_2 is the *appropriate respiratory compensation* for a metabolic acidosis.

TABLE 4-10. *COMPENSATORY CHANGES IN PRIMARY ACID–BASE DISORDERS*

CONDITION	PRIMARY CHANGE	EXPECTED COMPENSATION
Metabolic acidosis	$\downarrow HCO_3^-$	$\downarrow pCO_2 = 1.2 \times \downarrow [HCO_3^-]$
Metabolic alkalosis	$\uparrow HCO_3^-$	$\uparrow pCO_2 = 0.7 \times \uparrow [HCO_3^-]$
Respiratory acidosis		
Acute	$\uparrow pCO_2$	$\uparrow [HCO_3^-] = 0.1 \times \uparrow pCO_2$
Chronic	$\uparrow pCO_2$	$\uparrow [HCO_3^-] = 0.35 \times \uparrow pCO_2$
Respiratory alkalosis		
Acute	$\downarrow pCO_2$	$\downarrow HCO_3^- = 0.2 \times \downarrow pCO_2$
Chronic	$\downarrow pCO_2$	$\downarrow HCO_3^- = 0.4 \times \downarrow pCO_2$

$\downarrow$, decrease; $\uparrow$, increase.
(Adapted from Rose BD. Clinical physiology of acid-base and electrolyte disorders. 4th ed. New York, McGraw-Hill, 1994:508.)

PROBLEM 5

A patient in the intensive care unit with encephalitis had the following blood gas profile: pH, 7.50; pCO$_2$, 20 mm Hg; HCO$_3^-$, 14 mEq/L. What is the acid–base disorder? How should this patient be treated?

ANSWERS: The pH is increased, and the pCO$_2$ is decreased. This is a respiratory alkalosis secondary to central nervous system respiratory center stimulation. The condition must be relatively chronic, because there has been substantial renal compensation. The disorder itself should not be treated. In fact, the low pCO$_2$ may serve to partially counteract the cerebral edema. As this case demonstrates, it is important not to assume that any patient with a decreased HCO$_3^-$ has a metabolic acidosis.

PROBLEM 6

A 25-year-old patient with epilepsy suffered a grand mal seizure. Immediately after the seizure, the following laboratory values were obtained: arterial pH, 7.14; pCO$_2$, 45 mm Hg; HCO$_3^-$, 14 mEq/L; Na$^+$, 140 mEq/L; Cl$^-$, 98 mEq/L. What kind of acidosis is present? What is the anion gap, and why is it increased?

ANSWERS: This is a case of increased anion gap metabolic acidosis secondary to lactic acid production from skeletal muscles during tonic–clonic seizure activity. The anion gap is 140 mEq/L − (98 mEq/L + 17 mEq/L) = 25 mEq/L. There is also a respiratory acidosis due to depressed ventilation during the seizure.

MIXED ACID–BASE DISORDERS

Clinical problems are often complex; therefore, it is not unusual for patients to present with more than one concurrent acid–base disturbance (as in Problem 6). Such conditions are called mixed acid–base disorders and sometimes can be difficult to appreciate. However, with a good understanding of the processes by which the body reacts to acid–base disturbances, it is relatively easy to detect the simultaneous presence of two or three different disorders.

Mixed metabolic alkalosis and respiratory alkalosis can produce severe alkalemia. In this case, the pCO$_2$ is decreased, and the HCO$_3^-$ is increased, which will severely decrease the pCO$_2$-to-HCO$_3^-$ ratio and the H$^+$ concentration. A common cause of this mixed disorder is seen during the first trimester of pregnancy in women who have severe nausea and vomiting. Pregnancy is associated with a respiratory alkalosis normally, and if severe morning sickness ensues, a chloride-responsive contraction alkalosis will occur.

Mixed metabolic alkalosis and respiratory acidosis produces a high pCO$_2$ and a high HCO$_3^-$. A more normal pCO$_2$-to-HCO$_3^-$ ratio and pH are observed than would be predicted for either disorder alone. A common example of this condition is a patient with chronic obstructive pulmonary disease who develops a chloride-responsive metabolic alkalosis as a result of diuretic administration or other cause of volume contraction during an exacerbation of the lung disease or, alternatively, as a result of the administration of corticosteroids for treatment of the lung disease. In this setting, CO$_2$ retention may become more pronounced, because ventilation decreases to compensate for the metabolic alkalosis.

Mixed metabolic acidosis and respiratory acidosis can lower the pH to extremely low and dangerous levels. Patients with cardiopulmonary arrest invariably have mixed metabolic and respiratory acidoses until adequate ventilation is established.

Mixed metabolic acidosis and respiratory alkalosis occur reasonably frequently in critically ill patients and indicate a poor prognosis. Patients with hepatic insufficiency may manifest this combination. Such patients have baseline respiratory alkalosis and often develop metabolic acidosis as a result of sepsis and lactic acidosis or alcoholic ketoacidosis.

Mixed metabolic acidosis and metabolic alkalosis obviously offset one another and can be difficult to diagnose. Clues to their concurrence can be obtained from the patient history, the anion gap, and occasionally, the serum potassium. Many insulin-dependent diabetic patients have significant nausea and vomiting preceding a bout of diabetic ketoacidosis. The vomiting produces a chloride-responsive contraction alkalosis, and the ketoacidosis produces a high anion gap acidosis. Together, they can produce a relatively normal pH; however, the patient history and a very high anion gap show that something is awry. A similar but more difficult condition to diagnose occurs in patients with severe gastroenteritis manifested by both vomiting and diarrhea, causing alkalosis and a normal anion gap acidosis, respectively. In this case, the history may provide the only clue to diagnosis.

Triple acid–base disorders are combinations of metabolic acidosis, metabolic alkalosis, and a respiratory disorder. These disorders can be difficult to diagnose and require careful attention to the clinical history.

CASE 2

A 38-year-old male electrician with chronic glomerulonephritis had been followed by a medical house officer in the clinic at the university hospital for the past 3 years. Because the house officer is leaving the university, she asks an incoming intern to take over the care of this patient. On the first day of his internship, he is paged to the emergency room to see the patient. The patient complains of increasing shortness of breath and a productive cough. The patient has a temperature of 39°C and rales in his lower left posterior lung field, and he was tachypneic, with a respiratory rate of 22 breaths/minute. The emergency department resident says that the arterial blood gasses show that the patient is mildly hypoxic, but there is no significant acid–base disorder because the pH was normal. The new intern is somewhat perplexed by this diagnosis and asks to see the laboratory test values, which are as follows: blood urea nitrogen, 85 mg/dl; creatinine, 7.2 mg/dl; HCO_3^-, 12 mM; pH, 7.4; pCO_2, 20 mm Hg. Having just completed his renal rotation as a fourth-year medical student, the new intern knows exactly what was happening.

CASE DISCUSSION

This case illustrates the principle that when two counteracting acid–base disorders are present, the pH of the blood can be high, low, or normal. Because *compensatory processes do not return the pH to normal,* an equation or nomogram is not needed to diagnose a combined or mixed acid–base disorder in this case. The two counteracting disorders are metabolic acidosis and respiratory alkalosis. The metabolic acidosis is the result of chronic renal failure, and the respiratory alkalosis occurred because of the patient's pneumonia, which was confirmed by chest X-ray films. If this diagnosis seems confusing, individually consider the laboratory abnormalities: decreased HCO_3^- concentration and decreased pCO_2. If the decreased HCO_3^- concentration was the only primary change (i.e., if only a metabolic acidosis was present), the expected compensatory decrease in pCO_2 would be approximately 1.2 mm Hg for every 1-mM fall in $[HCO_3^-]$ = 1.2 mm Hg $\times$ (24 mm Hg − 14 mm Hg) = 12 mm Hg, or a decrease from 40 mm Hg to 28 mm Hg. Because the patient's actual pCO_2 level is considerably less than 28 mm Hg, it follows that there is some other primary stimulus for the decreased pCO_2. Conversely, if the decrease in pCO_2 was the only primary change (i.e., if only a metabolic acidosis was present), the expected compensatory decrease in HCO_3^- concentration would be 2 mM for every 10-mm Hg fall in PCO_2 if the respiratory alkalosis was acute, or 5 mEq/L for every 10-mm Hg fall in pCO_2 if the respiratory alkalosis was chronic. Therefore, the expected fall in HCO_3^- concentration would be 2 mM $\times$ 2 mM = 4 mM in acute respiratory alkalosis, and 2 mM $\times$ 5 mM = 10 mM in chronic respiratory alkalosis. Because the fall in HCO_3^- concentration is actually much greater than predicted, even if the respiratory alkalosis was chronic, which almost certainly it was not, this indicates that some other primary cause explained the decrease in HCO_3^- concentration.

PROBLEM 7

A patient has an arterial blood pH of 7.4 and a pCO_2 of 20 mm Hg.

    A. *What is the HCO_3^- concentration?*

    B. *What, if any, acid–base disorder(s) is/are present? Assume pH = 7.4 is normal.*

ANSWERS

    A. $[HCO_3^-] = 24 \times pCO_2/[H^+] = 24 \times 20/40 = 12$ mEq/L.

    B. Because pH is normal, because both the pCO_2 and the $[HCO_3^-]$ are abnormally low, and because normal compensatory processes do not completely correct the pH for an acid–base disorder, these data depict a patient with a combined metabolic acidosis and respiratory alkalosis.

PROBLEM 8

A previously well patient is brought to the emergency room in severe respiratory distress. Physical examination and chest X-ray films suggest acute pulmonary edema. Laboratory tests values are as follows:

arterial pH	7.02
pCO_2	60 mm Hg
HCO_3^-	15 mEq/L
pO_2	40 mm Hg
Cl^-	95 mEq/L
Na+	140 mEq/L

(continued)

A. *What acid–base disorder(s) is/are present?*
B. *Why is the HCO_3^- decreased?*

Answers

A. The blood is acidemic; therefore, at least one type of acidosis is present. The pCO_2 is high, and the $[HCO_3^-]$ is low, both of which would increase $[H^+]$. Neither of these changes could be compensatory. Therefore, this patient has combined metabolic and respiratory acidoses.

B. Although there is not enough clinical information presented to explain the cause of the metabolic acidosis, it is a high anion gap acidosis. The most likely explanation is lactic acidosis caused by anoxia and poor tissue perfusion in a patient with severe congestive heart failure and pulmonary edema.

Problem 9

A 24-year-old man with insulin-dependent diabetes mellitus develops symptoms of a viral infection. He is febrile, anorexic, and nauseated, and he has vomited several times in the 48-hour period before admission to the hospital. Because he was not eating, he took no long-lasting insulin the day previous to or the day of admission to the hospital. On admission, his laboratory test values are as follows:

arterial pH	7.36
pCO_2	35 mm Hg
HCO_3^-	20 mEq/L
Cl^-	90 mEq/L
Na^+	140 mEq/L
K^+	3.8 mEq/L

Is/are there any significant acid–base disorder(s) present? If so, which one(s)? How should this patient be treated?

Answers

A. This patient has severe ketoacidosis and a concurrent metabolic alkalosis caused by vomiting and volume contraction. The highly elevated anion gap (30 mEq/L) shows that substantial amounts of an unmeasured anion (i.e., ketones) are present. The fact that the anion gap is significantly greater than the change from normal in $[HCO_3^-]$ provides the major clue that two disorders are present. If untreated, this patient will become severely *acidemic* (i.e., blood pH will decrease) as well as acidotic within a few hours.

B. Because the patient is severely acidotic despite relatively normal blood pH and $[HCO_3^-]$, he should be aggressively treated like any patient with diabetic ketoacidosis—with volume replacement, intravenous insulin, potassium supplementation, and careful monitoring of blood sugar and anion gap.

SELECTED READING

Jacobson HR. Chloride-responsive metabolic alkalosis. In: Seldin DW, Giebisch G, eds. The kidney: physiology and pathophysiology. New York: Raven Press, 1988.

Narins RG, Emmett M. Simple and mixed acid–base disorders: a practical approach. Medicine 1980:59,161.

Lippincott's Pathophysiology Series: Renal Pathophysiology, edited by James A. Shayman. J. B. Lippincott Company, Philadelphia © 1995.

Proteinuria

David Kershaw
Roger C. Wiggins

OBJECTIVES

By the end of this chapter the reader should be able to:

- Describe the structure of the glomerulus and relate its structure to its function as a filter.
- State the factors that determine whether a protein is filtered or excluded.
- State the site and mechanism of tubular handling of filtered proteins.
- State the composition and amount of protein normally present in the urine.
- Describe the methods of measuring protein excretion in the urine.
- Describe functional and orthostatic proteinuria.
- Describe four major mechanisms that can cause pathologic proteinuria.
- List examples of renal diseases that can lead to each type of proteinuria.
- Define the nephrotic syndrome.
- Explain how renal biopsy can help in management of the nephrotic syndrome.
- Describe the supportive therapy used to treat the nephrotic syndrome.

The detection of protein on routine examination of the urine may be the first and only sign of serious renal disease, or it may reflect a minor, unimportant abnormality. Determining the importance and the underlying cause of the proteinuria requires an understanding of the physiology of renal protein handling and the pathophysiologic consequences of excessive loss of protein in the urine.

THE PHYSIOLOGY OF RENAL PROTEIN HANDLING

The kidneys of an average 70-kg adult have a blood flow of 1.1 L/minute (about 20% of cardiac output) and a plasma flow of 600 ml/minute. Each kidney of a normal adult contains about 1 million nephrons. The glomerulus of each nephron is a modified blood vessel whereby the afferent arteriole splits into 3 or 4 branches to form a tuft of capillary loops before rejoining to form the efferent arteriole by which blood exits the glomerulus. The filtrate of blood is formed by hydrostatic pressure working against oncotic pressure (i.e., Starling's forces) to drive the filtrate across the wall of the glomerular capillary loop. Angiotensin II causes efferent arteriolar constriction, thereby increasing the fraction of the blood that is filtered. The filtrate collects within Bowman's space before it travels down the renal tubule to be modified by reabsorption of substances the body will retain (e.g., water, ions, glucose) and secretion into the tubular fluid of waste products to be excreted. The amount of plasma filtered by both kidneys combined is 125 ml/minute, or 180 L/day, representing about 60 times the body's entire plasma volume. Under normal conditions, less than 150 mg of protein are excreted in the urine each day. Because 1 L of plasma contains 60 to 80 g of protein, this small amount of protein excreted demonstrates the extraordinary retention of proteins by the renal filtration mechanism.

PROBLEM 1

Calculate the fraction of the filtered protein load that is excreted by the kidneys each day.

ANSWER: The kidney filters approximately 180 L of plasma each day, containing about 70 g of protein/L. The protein load on the filter therefore is 12,600 g/day (180 L/day times 70 g/L). The normal upper limit for urinary protein excreted per day is 150 mg (0.15 g). Thus, the fraction of protein that is excreted is 0.15 g/12,600 g = 0.000012, or 0.001%.

STRUCTURE OF THE GLOMERULAR FILTER

The filtration surface consists of three layers, as illustrated in Figure 5-1.

Endothelium

On the inner surface of the filter in contact with blood is a fenestrated endothelium. Holes (fenestrae) about 70 nm in diameter traverse the body of the endothelial cell lining the inner aspect of the capillary to form the first part of the filtration barrier. These holes are a minimal barrier to plasma proteins, which are relatively much smaller than these holes; albumin and IgG molecules are 3.6 and 5.5 nm in diameter, respectively.

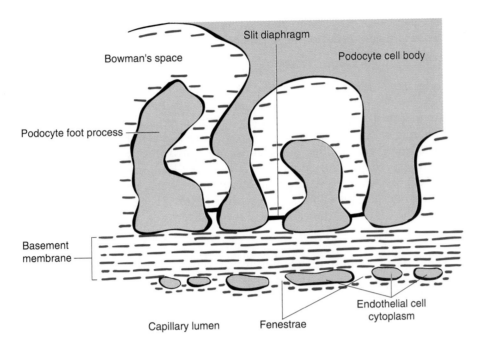

— Negatively charged molecules

Figure 5-1. The glomerular filtration surface showing the inner layer of fenestrated endothelium, the glomerular basement membrane, and the outer layer of podocyte foot processes between which the filtrate passes.

Glomerular Basement Membrane

The glomerular basement membrane (GBM) is a cell-free matrix about 300 nm thick composed of glycoproteins, including fibronectin, laminin, type IV collagen, and negatively charged heparan sulfate proteoglycans. GBM contains six different variants of type IV collagen chains, called α1 through α6 type IV collagen. Each chain is encoded by a different gene. The genes are arranged in pairs on three different chromosomes. At least two of the type IV collagen chains have important clinical syndromes associated with them; these are Alport's syndrome and Goodpasture's syndrome.

Alport's Syndrome. The α5 and α6 type IV collagen chains are located on the X chromosome. Mutations of the α5 type IV collagen gene cause Alport's syndrome (i.e., chronic hereditary nephritis), which is a clinical syndrome of renal failure, deafness, and lens abnormalities of the eye. In this condition, in which basement membranes in the glomerulus, cochlear, and lens disintegrate over time, males are more severely affected than females, because males have only one gene for α5 type IV collagen, whereas females have two. Thus, females can compensate for an abnormal α5 type IV collagen molecule, whereas males cannot.

Goodpasture's Syndrome. In individuals with the correct genetic background, autoantibodies may develop to the α3 type IV collagen chain. This results in immune-mediated attack on the GBM and lung basement membrane, which also have these collagen chains. The consequence of this immune attack on the GBM are inflammatory destruction of the glomerular capillary wall, leakage of blood into Bowman's space, impaired glomerular filtration, and acute renal failure; consequences in the lung are destruction of the alveolar wall, leakage of blood into alveolae, impaired gas exchange, and acute respiratory failure.

Glomerular Epithelial Cell (Podocyte)

Podocytes cover the outer aspect of the glomerular basement membrane. Podocytes have a main cell body and octopus-like tentacles that end in foot processes that project out to cover the whole filtration surface. The foot processes of neighboring cells interdigitate. Between the interdigitated foot processes, there are narrow slits (i.e., modified intercellular junctions) through which the filtrate passes. These slit diaphragms function as part of the filtration mechanism. The surface of adjacent foot processes are coated by negatively charged sialoglycoproteins. Thus, the glomerular filtration barrier consists of three layers: the fenestrated endothelium, the GBM, and the glomerular epithelial cell foot processes.

Mesangium and Mesangial Cells

The capillary loops of the glomerulus are supported like the foliage of a tree by a central core or trunk with branches. This trunk and its branches are composed of mesangial cells and mesangial matrix. Mesangial cells contract in response to angiotensin II and other mediators, thereby modifying access of blood to the filtration surface. They are also phagocytic and can remove and destroy immune complexes from blood that are trapped on the glomerular filter. Mesangial cells reside in a matrix of collagen, fibronectin, laminin, and other proteins. Injury to the glomerulus is often associated with an increase in the amount of this matrix, an increase in the number of cells in the mesangial compartment of the glomerulus, or both.

CHARACTERISTICS OF THE GLOMERULAR FILTER

Functionally, the glomerulus exhibits both size-selective and charge-selective filtration properties. Molecules with radii less than 2.5 nm (e.g., water, ions, glucose, urea) pass freely across the filter. As the molecular radius increases above 4 nm, filtration becomes restricted. Charge selectivity refers to the property of the glomerular filter that excludes negatively charged macromolecules more readily than neutral or positively charged macromolecules. This charge barrier is thought to arise from fixed negative charges present on the endothelium, basement membrane, and podocyte foot processes. Thus, the passage of the major plasma protein, albumin, which has a negative charge at physiologic pH (pI 4.6) and a molecular radius of about 3.6 nm, is impeded mostly on the basis of its charge and not on the basis of its size. The importance of the charge effect is emphasized by the fact that although the albumin molecule is small enough to pass through the filter, the ratio of concentration of albumin in plasma to its concentration in the glomerular filtrate is approximately 4000 to 1.

PROBLEM 2

There are two main forms of amylase that circulate in blood; these are pancreatic isoamylase and salivary isoamylase. These have a nearly identical molecular mass

(continued)

(slightly less than that of albumin), but they differ in effective charge at physiologic pH. The isoelectric point (pI) of pancreatic isoamylase is 7, and the pI of salivary isoamylase is 6. Predict the relative clearance of the two forms of amylase for a normal volunteer and for a patient who has lost the charge barrier but not the size barrier in their glomerular filter.

Answer: At physiologic pH (7.4) the salivary isoamylase (pI 6) has given up more of its protons than pancreatic isoamylase (pI 7) and thus has a greater net negative charge. Both isoamylases are partially retained on the basis of their size, but the salivary isoamylase is also impeded from passing through the filter because of its greater negative charge. Thus, the clearance from blood of pancreatic isoamylase is greater than that for salivary isoamylase. In patients with minimal-change nephrotic syndrome, the charge barrier but not the size barrier of the glomerulus is lost. Because the size of both forms of isoamylases are nearly identical, they should have similar clearances in this condition.

FILTERED PROTEINS APPEARING IN THE URINE

The protein excreted in the urine represents only a small fraction of the protein that is filtered. The bulk of the filtered protein is reabsorbed by the proximal convoluted tubule. Proteins are reabsorbed by endocytosis through the luminal cell membrane. Proteins, along with some tubular fluid, are pinched off in vesicles that form between the microvilli of the apical cell membrane. These vesicles fuse with other endocytotic vesicles and with cytoplasmic lysosomal vesicles that contain hydrolytic enzymes. The reabsorbed proteins are digested and returned to the body as amino acids or small peptides. The capacity of the proximal tubule to reabsorb individual proteins varies even for proteins of similar size and charge. The major low molecular-weight proteins present in normal urine that escape reabsorption are β_2-microglobulin, lysozyme, α_1-microglobulin, and α_2-microglobulin. For small plasma proteins, approximately 98% of the filtered load reaching the tubule is reabsorbed.

PROTEINS ORIGINATING IN THE URINARY TRACT

The urine contains proteins in addition to those filtered by the glomerulus. These proteins originate from the urinary tract and account for about 50% of urinary protein. Most of this protein is a large glycoprotein called Tamm-Horsfall protein (uromucoid). Tamm-Horsfall protein is secreted by the cells of the thick ascending limb of Henle and is the major protein component of urinary hyaline casts, which are found in normal urine. Waxy casts are broader and more refractive than hyaline casts and are not a component of normal urine. They are usually indicative of severe renal disease (Fig. 5-2). Other proteins of urogenital tract origin also may be found in normal urine. These include proteins from the ureters, bladder, urethra, accessory sex glands, and kidney. The amount of urogenital-tract–origin protein excreted in the urine may increase dramatically with infection, inflammation, or tumors of the urogenital tract. Normal urinary protein is composed of approximately 40% albumin, 10% IgG, 5% light chains, and 3% IgA. The remainder consists of other proteins, mostly Tamm-Horsfall protein.

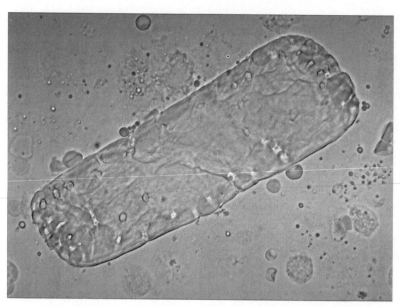

Figure 5-2. Waxy cast found in the urine of individuals with chronic renal failure and proteinuria and distinguished from a hyaline cast by its highly refractile appearance. (Picture reproduced with permission from Haber HM. Urine casts, their microscopy and clinical significance. Chicago: American Society of Clinical Pathologists, 1976.)

THE CLINICAL ASSESSMENT OF PROTEINURIA

DIPSTICK AND TURBIDITY TESTS

In normal clinical practice, a urine specimen is checked for protein by using a urinary dipstick. This colorometric test is based on the ability of proteins to alter the color of particular acid–base indicators independent of altering the pH. The test is more sensitive for albumin than for other proteins, particularly immunoglobulin light chains, which are found in monoclonal form in multiple myeloma. The commonly used scale of reporting results is: negative, <10 mg/dl; trace, 10 mg/dl; 1+, 30 mg/dl; 2+, 100 mg/dl; and 3+, >500 mg/dl. False-positive test results can occur when testing an alkaline urine (pH >8). Turbidity tests are also used to confirm the presence of proteinuria. Sulfosalicylic acid added to a urine specimen causes the proteins to precipitate. The resulting turbidity is then compared visually to a set of color standards and read on a 1-to-4+ scale. The turbidity tests are capable of detecting all proteins, but are prone to false-positives with some drugs (e.g., tolbutamide, some penicillin derivatives). Both the dipstick and turbidity methods give an estimate of urine protein concentration but do not necessarily accurately reflect the total urinary protein excretion.

PROBLEM 3

Consider the urine of two patients. Patient A excretes 450 ml of urine per day with a protein concentration of 30 mg/dl. Patient B excretes 3.5 L of urine per day with a protein concentration of 10 mg/dl. What is the degree of proteinuria exhibited by each patient?

(continued)

ANSWER: Patient A has a 24-hour urinary protein excretion of 135 mg, which is within normal limits, but he also has an abnormal dipstick reading of 1+. Patient B has a trace dipstick reading, which is within the normal range, but she has a 24-hour urine protein excretion of 350 mg, which is more than twice the upper limit of normal. A more accurate estimate of the leakiness of the glomerular filter would be to collect all urine passed during a complete day for each patient.

THE 24-HOUR URINE COLLECTION FOR PROTEIN

The normal 24-hour total protein excretion for adults is less than 150 mg. There is a normal diurnal variation in protein, with maximal excretions rates occurring during normal daily activities. This is related to the effects of ambulation and upright posture increasing hemodynamic forces on the glomerular filter.

Because of the limitations of the screening tests outlined in Problem 3, quantitative methods are commonly employed to assess protein excretion rate. A timed urine sample, typically over 24 hours, is collected and analyzed to assess protein excretion. To ensure that the collection is complete, the total amount of creatinine in the sample is also measured. Creatinine is formed by the metabolism of creatine phosphate from muscle. The amount of creatinine produced per day is related mainly to a person's muscle mass and, to a small extent, on their meat intake that day. Creatinine production is therefore fairly constant from day to day for each individual. The normal expected creatinine excretion rates are 20 to 25 mg/kg/day for men, and 15 to 20 mg/kg/day for women.

PROBLEM 4

A 24-hour urine collection from a 70-kg man contains 700 mg creatinine and 140 mg protein in a total volume of 690 ml. Does this patient have increased protein excretion in the urine?

ANSWER: This urine collection is probably incomplete. At least 1.4 g of creatinine (70 kg × 20 mg/kg/day for a man) would be expected in the sample. Only 700 mg of creatinine is present in the sample. Thus, the patient probably placed only about one half of the urine passed into the container for protein and creatinine measurement. If only one half of the urine contained 140 mg of protein, then a complete collection would have contained about 280 mg of protein. This result would be above the upper limit of normal and could indicate significant underlying renal disease.

URINE PROTEIN–CREATININE RATIO

A second method of quantitating urine protein uses a single spot specimen in which protein and creatinine concentrations are measured. Because the rate of creatinine excretion is fairly constant throughout the day regardless of changes in urine flow rate, the ratio of the protein concentration to the creatinine concentration is constant. This protein–creatinine ratio shows an excellent correlation with 24-hour urine protein collections and is much simpler to collect, especially in young children and infants. The protein–creatinine ratio should be <0.2 in normal urine; protein and creatinine concentrations are measured in mg/dl.

PROBLEM 5

A urine collection from a 2-year-old child has a protein concentration of 30 mg/dl (1+ on dipstick) and a creatinine concentration of 180 mg/dl. Is this child passing more protein in the urine than normal?

ANSWER: The protein–creatinine ratio is 0.17, which is within normal limits.

ORTHOSTATIC PROTEINURIA

In some healthy persons, especially adolescents and young adults, the normal increase in protein excretion upon assuming an upright posture and daily activity may be accentuated. Excretion of up to 2 g of protein per day may occur during normal daily activity, whereas protein excretion during normal recumbency at night is within normal limits. This is termed postural or orthostatic proteinuria, a normal variation that does not indicate renal disease.

FUNCTIONAL PROTEINURIA

Proteinuria may occur in patients with normal kidneys in association with hemodynamic stress caused by high fever, congestive heart failure, exposure to cold, or some acute medical illnesses. Strenuous exercise may also lead to proteinuria. This type of proteinuria is termed functional, and by definition, the proteinuria resolves after the precipitating event is over.

PROBLEM 6

An 18-year-old man is found to have proteinuria on a sports physical examination. There is no hematuria. He weighs 72 kg. On physical examination, he has normal blood pressure, is well developed, and has no edema. He is asked to collect timed, upright/ambient, and recumbent urine collections. The upright collection is labeled from 8:00 am to 10:00 pm and contains 672 mg of creatinine with 1000 mg of protein. The recumbent collection is labeled from 10:00 pm to 8:00 am and contains 690 mg of creatinine with 50 mg of protein.

Calculate the protein excretion rate for both collections and decide whether the urine collections were performed properly. Are these collections consistent with the diagnosis of orthostatic proteinuria?

ANSWER: This 72-kg man would be expected to excrete 20 to 25 mg/kg/day of creatinine in his urine, or about 1 mg/kg/hour. In his 8:00 am to 10:00 pm collection (14 hours), about 1000 mg of creatinine would be expected (672 mg measured). In his 10:00 pm to 8:00 am collection (10 hours) about 720 mg would be expected (690 mg measured). Therefore, it can be concluded that the 8:00 am to 10:00 pm collection is probably incomplete, because there is insufficient creatinine present. The 10:00 pm to 8:00 am collection appears adequate.

(continued)

By using the protein–creatinine ratios, it can be seen that the upright collection has a ratio of 1.48, whereas the recumbent collection has a ratio of 0.07, which is within the normal range of <0.2. Therefore, it can be concluded that the proteinuria in this case is orthostatic, and it is unlikely that there is serious underlying renal disease in this man.

USE OF URINE PROTEIN ELECTROPHORESIS IN THE CLASSIFICATION OF PROTEINURIA

Electrophoretic analysis of the proteins in urine is often useful for differentiating between the various forms of proteinuria. Two major strategies are used clinically. These are the simple separation of proteins according to their charge and size, and the specific identification of individual proteins using specific antibodies (i.e., immunoelectrophoresis or immunofixation).

URINE PROTEIN ELECTROPHORESIS (UPEP)

Urine proteins are separated on a support media by an applied electric current. At pH 8, negatively charged proteins (e.g., albumin) move rapidly toward the positively charged electrode. The proteins are visualized with a nonspecific protein stain. With this method, normal proteins in serum are separated into major peaks representing albumin, α_1-antitrypsin, α_2- macroglobulin, haptoglobulin, transferrin, C3 complement, and immunoglobulin. As shown in Figure 5-3, the patterns obtained by UPEP are typical for proteinuria of different types. UPEP can help determine if proteinuria is the result of a glomerular disorder, a tubular disorder, overload proteinuria, or a combination of these.

URINE IMMUNOELECTROPHORESIS (IEP)

Concentrated urine is placed in wells in a special gel and separated as in UPEP. After the proteins are separated, antisera to the proteins of interest are placed in wells between the lanes of the gel. The panel of antisera usually includes anti-IgG, anti-IgM, anti-IgA, anti-kappa, anti-lambda, and antipolyvalent. The antipolyvalent antiserum reacts with human immunoglobulins, including all light and heavy chain classes. The antibodies are allowed to diffuse onto the gel. Precipitation arcs form where the antibody and antigen complex. There are positive controls for each antigen tested. The urine IEP of the patient in Figure 5-3E shows the presence of free monoclonal lambda light chains consistent with the diagnosis of a light chain monoclonal gammopathy.

MECHANISMS OF PATHOLOGIC PROTEINURIA

Diseases that cause proteinuria usually do so through one of four major mechanisms (Fig. 5-4). The first two mechanisms relate to changes in the glomerular filtration barrier, resulting in the loss of the charge or size barrier of the glomerular filter. The third mechanism is based on the presence of abnormally high amounts of certain proteins in the plasma overwhelming the tubules' capacity to reabsorb the filtered protein (i.e., overload proteinuria). The fourth mechanism

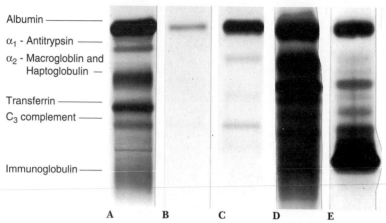

Albumin

α₁ - Antitrypsin

α₂ - Macrogloblin and Haptoglobulin

Transferrin

C₃ complement

Immunoglobulin

A B C D E

Figure 5-3. Urine protein electrophoresis (UPEP). (**A**) The serum protein electrophoresis (SPEP) pattern for normal human serum diluted 1 to 4. For UPEP, the urinary proteins must first be concentrated, because the protein concentration of the urine is often too small to be detected. (**B**) The usual pattern on UPEP for normal concentrated urine consists of a band for albumin. (**C**) Selective glomerular proteinuria shows a pattern on UPEP of albumin, α₁-antitypsin, and transferrin. Tubular proteinuria shows a pattern on UPEP of albumin, α₂-microglobulin, and β₂-microglobulin, seen between the transferrin and the C3 complement bands. (**D**) In many patients with proteinuria, there is a combination of glomerular and tubular dysfunction. Overload proteinuria shows a pattern on UPEP that is dependent on the specific protein in excess that is being filtered. (**E**) UPEP from a patient with a light chain monoclonal gammopathy showing a major band in the immunoglobulin region.

occurs when the ability of the proximal tubule to reabsorb protein is reduced. Loss of large quantities of protein in the urine (>3 g/day) almost always occurs in association with loss of the charge or size barrier of the glomerular filter and leads to the *nephrotic syndrome.* Thus, the amount of protein in the urine is also a useful indicator of the underlying mechanism involved.

LOSS OF THE CHARGE BARRIER AS A CAUSE OF PROTEINURIA

The charge barrier functions to exclude proteins with negative charges from crossing the glomerular filter. For albumin, a protein with pI 4.6 and radius of 3.5 nm, the loss of the charge barrier results in massive proteinuria, because the remaining size restriction of the filter is greater than the diameter of the albumin molecule. Transferrin (4 nm) also crosses, but IgG (5.5 nm) does not. The nature of the glomerular filtration defect can be determined clinically by measuring the ratio of IgG to transferrin in the urine. A low ratio of IgG to transferrin (<0.1) indicates a relatively specific loss of transferrin (i.e., albumin-like), suggesting that the charge barrier alone is defective. This is termed selective proteinuria and is associated with minimal-change nephropathy (MCNS), particularly in children.

The anatomic counterpart of functional loss of the charge barrier is loss of the delicately interdigitating foot processes of the podocyte. By transmission electron microscopy, this foot process effacement appears as though foot processes have fused to form a single continuous sheet of cytoplasm overlying the GBM, hence the term foot process fusion to describe this phenomenon. In MCNS the only anatomic abnormality corresponding to the loss of the charge barrier is foot process fusion as seen on electron microscopy over the whole surface of the

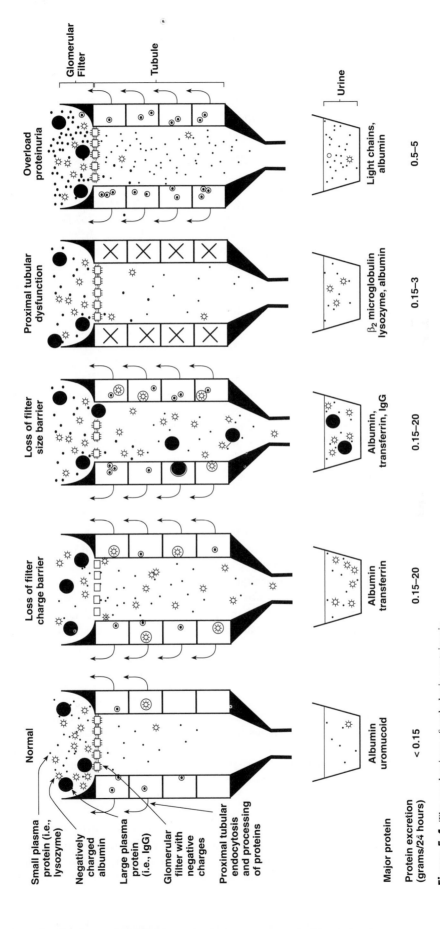

Figure 5-4. The mechanisms of pathologic proteinuria.

glomerular filter (i.e., diffuse distribution). Patchy or focal foot process fusion can be seen in many glomerular diseases associated with proteinuria and loss of the size barrier of the glomerular filter.

MINIMAL CHANGE NEPHROTIC SYNDROME

The features of MCNS are: (1) diffuse foot process fusion identified by electron microscopy; (2) a normal light microscopic appearance of glomeruli; (3) massive loss of protein in the urine; (4) selective proteinuria; (5) occurrence in more than 90% of children 1 to 6 years of age but only 10% of adults with nephrotic syndrome; (6) response to glucocorticoid therapy. The etiology of MCNS is unknown, but T-cell dysfunction may play a role. MCNS is often precipitated or exacerbated by infections, allergic reactions, and immunizations and can occur as a secondary phenomena in patients with lymphomas or Hodgkin's disease. Many of the drugs used to treat MCNS act on the immune system. The first-line treatment of MCNS is glucocorticoids. Ninety percent of patients will remit within 8 weeks of therapy, many within the first week. For those who frequently relapse or who do not respond to treatment with glucocorticoids, cytotoxic agents (e.g., cyclophosphamide, chlorambucil) or other immunosuppressive agents (e.g., cyclosporin, levamisole) are effective in some individuals. Those that do not respond frequently have patchy (segmental) scarring in some (focal) glomeruli and nonselective proteinuria (i.e., loss of size barrier). This type of scarring may progress to end-stage renal disease (ESRD) over months to years and is called *focal segmental glomerulosclerosis* (FSGS).

CASE 1

A 2-year-old boy is brought to the physician by his mother with a history of an upper respiratory tract infection for the past week and puffy eyelids for the past 2 days. He is afebrile, and blood pressure is normal. On examination, there is bilateral periorbital edema without pedal edema. The abdomen appears distended but is not tender to palpation, and no organomegaly is detected. The remainder of the physical examination is normal except for a clear nasal discharge. What should the next diagnostic step be?

CASE DISCUSSION

The crucial test here is simple urinalysis by dipstick. This will indicate if proteinuria is the underlying cause of periorbital edema and possible ascites. If the urine dipstick shows 3+ protein, then the patient probably has nephrotic or nephritic syndrome. If there is no blood in the urine, then the condition is most likely to be MCNS. On the other hand, if there is blood present, and urine microscopy shows red cell casts, then the likely cause is postinfectious glomerulonephritis.

Urinalysis in this case reveals 4+ protein with a negative dipstick test for blood. Microscopic examination shows only an occasional hyaline cast. The patient has a decreased serum albumin concentration of 2.4 g/dl (normal,

3.5-5 g/dl), a normal blood urea nitrogen and creatinine for age, and a raised blood cholesterol level. Therefore, this boy meets the criteria for a clinical diagnosis of nephrotic syndrome (ie., proteinuria, hypoproteinemia, edema, and hyperlipidemia). The absence of red blood cells in the urine makes MCNS the most likely underlying pathologic diagnosis. The child is treated with prednisone. The edema and proteinuria resolve after 2 weeks. Six months later, he relapses and again has a good response to prednisone. What is this child's long-term renal prognosis?

This child has steroid-responsive nephrotic syndrome. On the basis of this child's age, lack of hematuria or hypertension, and response to steroids, he probably has MCNS, and his long-term renal prognosis is excellent. No renal biopsy is necessary. If a renal biopsy is done, the electron microscopy would show foot process effacement (i.e., fusion) with an essentially normal light microscopic appearance (Fig. 5-5).

CASE 2

An 8-year-old boy presents with 3+ ankle edema and is found to have hypertension, hematuria, and 4+ proteinuria. A 24-hour urine collection contains 12 g of protein, and his serum albumin is 1.7 g/dl. Creatinine clearance is

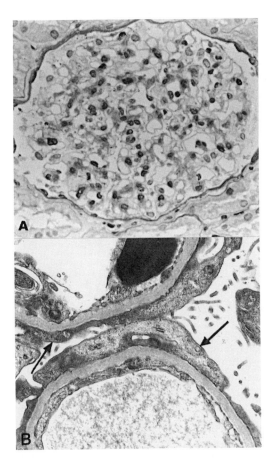

Figure 5-5. (A) Absence of abnormalities in glomerular capillary loops (× 400). (B) Electron microscopy (× 11,000) showing foot process effacement (*arrows*). Minimal-change nephropathy syndrome pathology. (From Knutson DW; Abt AB. Immune-mediated glomerulopathies. In: Kelley WN ed. Textbook of internal medicine. 2nd ed. Philadelphia: JB Lippincott; 1992:709.)

normal for his age. Laboratory tests for systemic lupus erythematosus, recent streptococcal infection, hepatitis B and C, and HIV are negative. He is treated with an 8- week course of daily prednisone without response. What is the next appropriate diagnostic or therapeutic step?

CASE DISCUSSION

A renal biopsy specimen will be helpful to assess therapy and prognosis in this case. The biopsy specimen shows patchy areas of scarring in some glomeruli consistent with a pathologic diagnosis of focal segmental glomerulosclerosis (FSGS) (Fig. 5-6). He is treated with a 12-week course of cyclophosphamide without response. Treatment with cyclosporine is associated with a reduction in 24-hour urine protein excretion to 3 g with improvement in his serum albumin and in his nephrotic symptoms. He relapses twice more when cyclosporine is discontinued. He is presently dependent on cyclosporine and antihypertensive agents for maintenance of his partial remission from nephrotic syndrome. It is unclear what the long-term prognosis will be, but he may progress to end-stage renal disease requiring dialysis and/or transplantation.

LOSS OF THE SIZE BARRIER IN THE GLOMERULAR FILTER

Many glomerular diseases cause nephrotic syndrome with loss of the size barrier. There is usually also patchy loss of the charge barrier in these glomeruli. In these diseases, the urine contains IgG as well as transferrin and albumin. The ratio of IgG to transferrin is greater than 0.1, and the proteinuria is termed nonselective. In general, the size barrier is lost and the glomerular filter leaks if:

Proteins accumulate in the filter wall (e.g., immune deposits containing IgG and C3 in immune complex disease; light chain, heavy chain, or serum

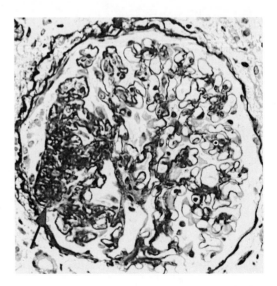

Figure 5-6. Focal segmental glomerulosclerosis pathology. A segmental area of sclerosis adhering to Bowman's capsule (*arrow*). (From Knutson DW; Abt AB. Immune-mediated glomerulopathies. In: Kelley WN ed. Textbook of internal medicine. 2nd ed. Philadelphia: JB Lippincott; 1992:709.)

amyloid deposits in different types of amyloidosis; increased amounts of extracellular matrix proteins in diabetes mellitus or FSGS).

Inflammatory cells are activated in the glomerular capillary wall and cause damage to the filter through release of proteolytic enzyme and oxidants (e.g., immune complex diseases caused by systemic lupus erythematosus, cryoglobulins, chronic infections, neoplasm).

CASE 3

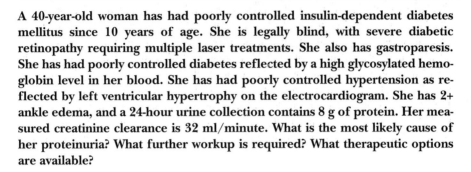

A 40-year-old woman has had poorly controlled insulin-dependent diabetes mellitus since 10 years of age. She is legally blind, with severe diabetic retinopathy requiring multiple laser treatments. She also has gastroparesis. She has had poorly controlled diabetes reflected by a high glycosylated hemoglobin level in her blood. She has had poorly controlled hypertension as reflected by left ventricular hypertrophy on the electrocardiogram. She has 2+ ankle edema, and a 24-hour urine collection contains 8 g of protein. Her measured creatinine clearance is 32 ml/minute. What is the most likely cause of her proteinuria? What further workup is required? What therapeutic options are available?

CASE DISCUSSION

The patient almost certainly has diabetic glomerulosclerosis (Kimmelstiel-Wilson lesions) with the nephrotic syndrome. There is no evidence of lupus or other systemic disease, although a foot ulcer with underlying osteomyelitis should be looked for in this woman with long-standing diabetes. Such a chronically infected ulcer could cause an immune complex disease or amyloidosis. Assuming that such an ulcer is excluded, no further diagnostic procedures are required. The most important therapeutic factors are control of her diabetes with insulin injections 3 to 4 times per day or an insulin pump and treatment of her hypertension with angiotensin-converting enzyme inhibitors and other agents as needed to a level of about 120/80 mm Hg. These therapeutic measures will slow the rate of progression of her renal failure; however, in the long term, her renal prognosis is poor, and it is likely she will progress to end-stage renal disease within 2 years. She therefore will require very careful follow-up with advice and planning regarding dialysis and/or renal transplantation.

CASE 4

A 23-year-old woman complains of arthralgias, fatigue, and increased sensitivity to the sun. Physical examination reveals a rash over her nose and cheeks. She states that for the past 2 years she has had intensely cold, painful hands during the winter. Her temperature is elevated at 39°C. Her blood pressure is elevated at 150/100 mm Hg. She has 1+ pedal edema. Dipstick urinalysis reveals 2+ protein and 1+ blood. Urine microscopy shows 15 white blood cells and 30 red blood cells per high power field. Granular and red blood cell

casts are present. Her serum creatinine is 1.5 mg/dl. What is the cause of this woman's proteinuria?

CASE DISCUSSION

This patient has a systemic disease which, from the clinical history and physical examination, is most likely an acute flare of systemic lupus erythematosus. Her urinalysis reveals evidence of acute inflammation of glomeruli (i.e., glomerulonephritis), including white blood cells in the urine, hematuria, proteinuria, and red blood cell casts. The granular casts and increased serum creatinine suggests that the inflammation is severe enough to interfere with renal function. Urgent treatment with glucocorticoids is required to prevent permanent loss of renal function. In this case, the proteinuria is a reflection of glomerular inflammation with loss of charge and size barrier as a result of immune complex–induced inflammation within the glomerular filter.

CASE 5

A 62-year-old man on no medications presents with ankle edema and recent-onset hypertension. Physical examination shows no abnormality except for 2+ pedal edema and a blood pressure of 160/100 mm Hg. Urinalysis shows 3+ protein, and 1+ blood, with occasional granular casts seen on urine microscopy. His 24-hour urine collection has 8 g of protein, and his creatinine clearance is 92 ml/minute. Blood studies show no evidence of diabetes or systemic lupus erythematosus. A cystoscopy, flat plate of the abdomen, and computed tomographic scan reveal no masses, stones, bladder problems, or prostate problems. What is the next step in his diagnostic workup?

CASE DISCUSSION

At this stage, a renal biopsy is needed to direct possible specific therapy for nephrotic syndrome. A renal biopsy shows subepithelial deposits of IgG and C3 and capillary loop thickening diagnostic of membranous nephropathy (Fig. 5-7). He is treated with 120 mg of prednisone on alternate days for 2 months. He is also treated with antihypertensive medication and diuretics. After 6 months of follow-up, his proteinuria has decreased to 500 mg/24 hours. On follow-up at 1 year, he has 2+ protein on dipstick, and he is asymptomatic with stable renal function and taking only a thiazide diuretic for mild hypertension.

This patient is one of approximately 25% to 50% who will remit from their idiopathic membranous nephropathy, either spontaneously or with treatment. In patients with secondary membranous nephropathy, who account for approximately one third of patients with membranous nephropathy, treatment consists of treatment of the underlying disease. In the over-60-year age group, about 10% of membranous nephropathy is associated with malignancy.

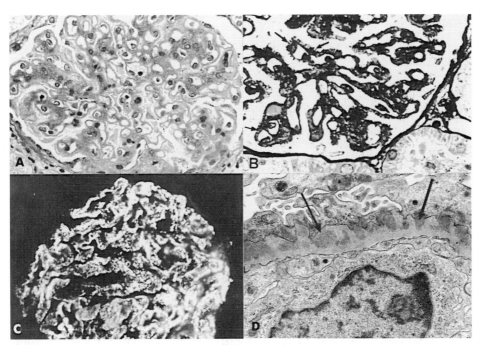

Figure 5-7. Membranous pathology. (**A**) Thickened capillary membranes throughout the glomerular tuft. (**B**) Silver methenamine stain revealing epimembranous spikes (*arrows*). (**C**) Granular deposits of IgG along glomerular capillary loops. (**D**) Electron micrograph (× 12,000). (From Knutson DW; Abt AB. Immune-mediated glomerulopathies. In: Kelley WN ed. Textbook of internal medicine. 2nd ed. Philadelphia: JB Lippincott; 1992:710.)

OVERLOAD PROTEINURIA

Overload proteinuria occurs when the plasma concentration of a small protein that normally would cross the filter to be reabsorbed in the proximal tubule is increased to the point where the filtered load of protein overwhelms the proximal tubules' ability to reabsorb the protein. Some of that protein ends up in the urine in abnormally high amounts. Three common proteins can cause overload proteinuria.

Light Chains

In some plasma cell disorders (e.g., multiple myeloma), increased synthesis of light chains by an uncontrolled clone of light chain–producing plasma cells results in increased concentration of light chains in the plasma and increased excretion of light chains into the urine. The light chains may precipitate in the tubule or cause tubule dysfunction by other mechanisms, thereby causing renal dysfunction along with proteinuria. Large amounts of light chains can be detected by heating a urine sample to 56°C and observing protein precipitation, followed by solubilization of the protein as the urine is heated to 100°C. This phenomenon is called Bence Jones proteinuria. This test is no longer routinely used. Immunoelectrophoresis is used to detect these monoclonal light chains in urine. The urine dipsticks used in the clinic are relatively insensitive to light chains, and a negative dipstick protein does not exclude light chains from being present in the urine.

Hemoglobin

Hemolysis sufficient to saturate the hemoglobin-binding protein (i.e., haptoglobin) in the blood results in hemoglobin appearing in the urine. Urine dipsticks are extremely sensitive to hemoglobin, and the presence of a positive urine dipstick for hemoglobin or blood without red cells being detectable by urine microscopy suggests hemolysis or rhabdomyolysis.

Myoglobin

When muscle tissue breaks down (i.e., rhabdomyolysis), myoglobin is released from muscle cells and can appear in the urine. Myoglobin is a heme pigment contained in a globulin chain that is about one fourth the size of hemoglobin and is easily filtered. Myoglobin in the urine gives a positive dipstick reading for hemoglobin. Myoglobinuria is suggested by a positive dipstick for hemoglobin or blood without red cells seen on microscopy.

CASE 6

A 60-year-old woman presents with complaints of weakness, fatigue, and weight loss. She had a bacterial pneumonia 6 weeks before this examination and has a recent history of back pain. Physical examination shows a pale woman who is clinically anemic. Her urinalysis shows trace protein on dipstick, with 3+ protein when assayed by sulfosalicylic acid turbidity. What diagnosis is suggested by her presentation and urinalysis?

CASE DISCUSSION

The clinical history is nonspecific, but in the context of a urinalysis suggesting nonalbumin proteinuria together with the anemia and recent onset of back pain, the diagnosis of multiple myeloma must be excluded. Laboratory tests show that the woman has anemia, mild hypercalcemia, and abnormal renal function (serum creatinine, 1.6 mg/dl). X-ray films of her lumbar spine show a collapsed L4 vertebra. Urine immunoelectrophoresis shows monoclonal lambda light chains. A bone marrow biopsy shows increased plasma cells. She meets criteria for a diagnosis of multiple myeloma, and therapy should be begun for this condition.

CASE 7

A 23-year-old man involved in a motor vehicle accident complains of diffuse abdominal pain. His urine is red, and it is found to have 4+ hematuria and 1+ proteinuria on dipstick analysis. There are more than 500 red blood cells per high power field on urine microscopy. What is the likely mechanism for the protein in the urine?

CASE DISCUSSION

The mechanism of this patient's proteinuria is bleeding caused by trauma to the urinary tract. The proteinuria is nonglomerular in origin. Blood, which contains 60 to 80 g of protein/L can leak into the urine because of trauma, renal calculi, infection, or tumors of the genitourinary system. This leads to a strongly positive test for hemoglobin and a positive test for protein on dipstick, with very large numbers of red blood cells seen on urine microscopic examination.

CASE 8

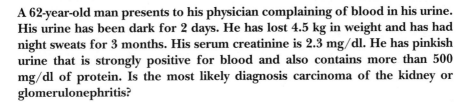

A 62-year-old man presents to his physician complaining of blood in his urine. His urine has been dark for 2 days. He has lost 4.5 kg in weight and has had night sweats for 3 months. His serum creatinine is 2.3 mg/dl. He has pinkish urine that is strongly positive for blood and also contains more than 500 mg/dl of protein. Is the most likely diagnosis carcinoma of the kidney or glomerulonephritis?

CASE DISCUSSION

The symptoms of weight loss and night sweats associated with hematuria could reflect either carcinoma of the kidney or systemic disease with glomerular involvement. How does the urine dipstick test help to distinguish between these possibilities? The finding of more than 500 mg/dl of protein on dipstick test suggests that there is more protein than would be expected by leakage of blood into the urinary tract alone, as would be the case for a renal cell carcinoma. A urocrit, which is similar to a hematocrit, can be measured. For there to be 500 mg/dl of protein, the urine the urocrit would have to be about 5%. Normal blood contains 50% hematocrit and 7 g/dl of protein; therefore, blood diluted 10% would contain 5% hematocrit and contain about 700 mg/dl protein. Ten percent blood is dark red; therefore, in this case there is more protein than can be expected by blood alone. The key investigation is urine microscopy, which shows red cell casts, granular casts, and 20 white blood cells per high power field, which confirms that there is inflammation in the glomeruli (i.e., glomerulonephritis), suggesting that vasculitis is the likely underlying pathologic process.

PROXIMAL TUBULE DYSFUNCTION CAUSING PROTEINURIA

Abnormal proximal tubular function for any reason may prevent the reabsorption of filtered proteins from the tubular lumen. The causes of tubular proteinuria may include primary renal diseases (e.g., tubulo interstitial diseases of congenital origin, Balkan nephropathy), side effects of drugs and toxins (e.g., heavy metal toxicity, analgesic nephropathy, ifosfamide toxicity), immune processes (e.g., transplant rejection, allergic interstitial nephritis), infection (e.g., CMV), and other systemic diseases (e.g., sickle cell anemia). Protein excretion is always less than 3 g/24 hours. The urinary proteins are limited to those proteins that normally cross the intact glomerular filtration barrier or are produced in the urinary tract. Albumin is present in the urine in tubulointerstitial diseases but at a much lower concentration relative to other smaller proteins than in diseases associated with a loss of the glomerular size or charge barrier. There may be other associated proximal tubular abnormalities such as a failure to reabsorb glucose, bicarbonate, phosphate, amino acids, and potassium. This broad spectrum of tubular abnormalities is called Fanconi's syndrome.

A 46-year-old man presents to the emergency room with gout. He is hypertensive, with a blood pressure of 160/105 mm Hg, and he has proteinuria of 2+ on dipstick with no blood in the urine. Additional tests show that he has a urine protein–creatinine ratio of 2.1 (normal, <0.2), and UPEP shows a tubular pattern of proteinuria. His serum creatinine concentration is 1.8 mg/dl, and his serum uric acid concentration is 8.5 mg/dl. Further questioning reveals that he has a long history of drinking home-distilled alcohol made from various fermented grains. How might this be related to his current medical problem?

CASE DISCUSSION

Hypertension itself can cause renal injury and proteinuria that is usually glomerular in type. Distillation of alcohol in the home is often done in old radiators or other homemade devices in which lead can gain access to the distillate from solder containing lead in the joints. The history is compatible with lead poisoning. Chronic lead poisoning in the adult can present as gout, hypertension, and renal failure caused by tubulointerstitial disease. A careful additional history and testing for lead poisoning will be useful.

NEPHROTIC SYNDROME

The nephrotic syndrome refers to a collection of diseases that share the cardinal features of *proteinuria* (>3 g/24 hours or a spot urine protein–creatinine ratio >3.5), *hypoproteinemia, edema, and hyperlipidemia.*

CAUSES

It is convenient to classify causes of the nephrotic syndrome into those that primarily affect only the kidney (i.e., primary renal diseases) and those that affect other organs as well (i.e., systemic renal diseases). Examples of primary renal diseases causing nephrotic syndrome include MCNS, idiopathic membranous nephropathy, membranoproliferative glomerulonephritis (MPGN), and congenital nephrotic syndrome. Examples of systemic disease associated with nephrotic syndrome include diabetic glomerulosclerosis; systemic lupus erthymatosus (SLE); other immune complex diseases caused by chronic infection (e.g., hepatitis B and C, malaria, syphilis, subacute bacterial endocarditis, shunt and intravenous line infections, abscesses); neoplasm; Henoch-Schönlein purpura; cirrhosis; pregnancy; drugs (e.g., penicillamine, gold, street heroin); amyloidosis caused by chronic infection, light chain deposition, or hereditary factors, and acquired immunodeficiency syndrome.

Children and adults differ in the prevalence of the etiologies of nephrotic syndrome, as shown in Table 5-1. The prevalence also varies among different countries and sites. For example, in nonindustrialized nations, hepatitis B infection and

TABLE 5-1. *CAUSES OF THE NEPHROTIC SYNDROME IN WESTERN COUNTRIES*		
	CHILDREN (%)	**ADULTS (%)**
Primary renal		
Minimal-change nephrotic syndrome	70	10
Other (e.g., membranous glomerulo-nephritis; membranoproliferative glomerulonephritis, focal glomerulo-sclerosis)	25	40
Secondary causes		
Diabetes mellitus		25
Collagen vascular disease (e.g., systemic lupus erythematosus, vasculitis)	5	15
Other (e.g., infection; neoplasm; acquired immunodeficiency syndrome; amyloidosis; drugs (such as gold, captopril, or penicillamine)		10

malaria are common causes of nephrotic syndrome in children. In inner cities, street heroin is a common cause of nephrotic syndrome in adults.

SIGNS AND SYMPTOMS

The patient may note frothy urine as the first sign of proteinuria as a result of the effect of protein in lowering the surface tension in the urine, as occurs when egg whites are beaten in a bowl. Because hypoproteinemia develops as a consequence of protein lost in the urine, edema may occur. In children, edema is usually first noted in the periorbital region and is often mistaken for an allergic reaction. Edema may also occur in the pleural and peritoneal cavities, scrotal or labial regions, and joints. In adults, edema is most often first noticed in the lower extremities if the person is ambulant during the day, and in the presacral region if the person is bed-bound during the day. Edema fluid is often redistributed and excreted as increased urine volume at night (i.e., nocturia).

The edema formation in the nephrotic syndrome is the result of excess salt and water reabsorption by the kidney. A simplified model of increased salt and water resorption in the nephrotic syndrome is shown in Figure 5-8. Salt and water retention is the result of a combination of autonomic and peptide reflexes triggered by the relative hypovolemia and decreased plasma oncotic pressure in the kidney that result from massive protein loss in the urine.

Hyperlipidemia occurs as a result of increased lipid production by the liver. This may contribute to long-term morbidity and mortality in patients with nephrotic syndrome by increasing their cardiovascular risk factors.

Aside from the presence of large amounts of protein in the urine (3–4+ protein), urinary findings in nephrotic syndrome also include oval fat bodies. Oval fat bodies are proximal tubular cells that have accumulated lipid by reabsorption from

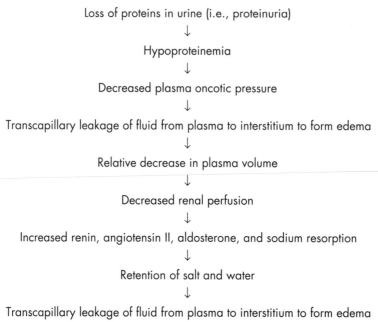

Figure 5-8. Mechanisms for increased salt and water retention in nephrotic syndrome. Other mechanisms such as vasopressin release, decreased atrial natriuretic factor release, and intrarenal mechanisms, also contribute.

the tubular lumen. These cells become detached from the tubular basement membrane and appear in the urine of individuals with large amounts of protein in their urine. Casts in the urine of people with proteinuria may also contain lipid and be granular (cell debris) or cellular, depending on the associated tubular and glomerular damage. Hematuria and hypertension frequently occur in glomerular diseases associated with nephrotic syndrome, with the exception of MCNS.

COMPLICATIONS

Complications of the nephrotic syndrome include *hyperlipidemia,* which over long periods of time may predispose to increased atherosclerosis, particularly in association with hypertension, which is common in individuals with glomerular diseases. There is an increased susceptibility to *infection* in nephrotic syndrome, especially by encapsulated organisms such as the pneumococcus. This may be due to the loss of immunoglobulins in the urine. *Thrombosis* is common in individuals with the nephrotic syndrome, leading to deep venous thromboses in the legs, renal vein thrombosis, or pulmonary emboli. This tendency of the blood to clot is partially explained by the urinary loss of antithrombin III and other inhibitors and regulators of coagulation. The *metabolism of drugs* carried by proteins may be abnormal. The *measurement of hormones* carried by protein in blood is abnormal (e.g., thyroid hormones).

TREATMENT

Therapy of the nephrotic syndrome can be divided into specific therapy for a particular disease causing the nephrotic syndrome and nonspecific general measures that can be applied to any person with the nephrotic syndrome, regardless of the underlying cause.

Specific Therapy

Childhood nephrotic syndrome can usually be assumed to be MCNS if the age, history, and laboratory findings are consistent with the diagnosis. Initial specific treatment of MCNS is daily corticosteroids for 8 to 12 weeks. Failure to respond to a course of glucocorticoids necessitates that a definitive diagnosis be reached by using a renal biopsy specimen to define the pathologic diagnosis and guide therapeutic decision-making.

Adult nephrotic syndrome has a variety of causes that may require specific therapies. For example, immunosuppression in an individual with lupus nephritis or excellent control of diabetes has been shown to reduce the rate of complications. Unless the cause is obvious (e.g., diabetes mellitus) a pathologic diagnosis by renal biopsy is often necessary. In specific conditions, use of corticosteroids, cytotoxic agents (e.g., cyclophosphamide), and other immunosuppressive agents (e.g., cyclosporin A) are useful. In some cases of idiopathic nephrotic syndrome, a trial of glucocorticoid therapy for up to 12 weeks may be a preferred therapeutic strategy prior to renal biopsy if there are no contraindications for steroid treatment in that individual. If this strategy is followed and there is no response to corticosteroids, then a renal biopsy for diagnostic, prognostic, and therapeutic decision-making purposes can be performed at a later stage.

Nonspecific Therapy

General behavior to maintain good health (e.g., exercise, moderate protein intake, low cholesterol diet, optimal weight control, no smoking) assume additional importance in patients with the nephrotic syndrome because of the secondary effects of the syndrome (e.g., hypertension, hyperlipidemia) and the side effects of drugs given to treat nephrotic syndrome (e.g., glucocorticoid side effects causing hypertension, hyperlipidemia, weight gain, increased appetite). Patients with nephrotic syndrome have a tendency to retain salt and water; therefore, a low-salt diet is prescribed to minimize fluid accumulation. When excessive extravascular fluid accumulates (i.e., edema), diuretics are often necessary to promote sodium and water excretion. Diuretics must be used judiciously in these patients, because excessive diuresis will cause intravascular volume depletion and increase the risk of hypoperfusion of the kidney and thrombosis. Thigh-high elastic stockings may help prevent fluid accumulation in the lower extremities during ambulation.

Angiotensin converting enzyme (ACE) inhibitors can reduce protein loss in the urine by reducing intraglomerular pressure and GFR. This reduction in protein loss, reduction in intraglomerular pressure, and inhibition of angiotensin II effects may also be helpful in reducing fluid retention in the nephrotic syndrome. ACE inhibitors have been shown to reduce the rate of loss of renal function in diabetic glomerulosclerosis by 50%. Similar protective effects may be anticipated in many forms of glomerular diseases associated with the nephrotic syndrome. Data from controlled trials for these conditions are not yet available.

Treatment of systemic hypertension is essential in nephrotic syndrome. Patients with nephrotic syndrome often have hypertension as a result of the renal or systemic disease causing the nephrotic syndrome. Hypertension is also a side effect of some of the drugs used to treat nephrotic syndrome (especially glucocorticoids). It is important to effectively reduce hypertension to normal or low-normal levels in patients with nephrotic syndrome to prevent both the acute complications (e.g., seizures, heart failure, encephalopathy) and chronic complications (e.g., accelerated loss of renal function, atherosclerosis, heart disease, stroke) of hypertension. ACE inhibitors are first-line drugs for this purpose for the reasons outlined previously.

If the nephrotic syndrome is very severe, it may be necessary to reduce the loss of protein by reducing the GFR pharmacologically by use of nonsteroidal anti-inflammatory agents, ACE inhibitors, or both, in association with high-dose diuretics. It may sometimes be helpful to remove fluid by infusions of salt-poor albumin to increase plasma oncotic pressure and plasma volume, combined with intravenous diuretic therapy to mobilize fluid from the tissues. In rare cases, it may be necessary to remove fluid by extracorporeal ultrafiltration. In extreme cases, such as in *congenital nephrotic syndrome* affecting very young children, bilateral nephrectomy may be required to prevent complications from the massive, life-threatening protein loss in the urine. In this case, the person would be maintained on dialysis pending renal transplantation.

CASE 10

A 56-year-old man with long-standing hypertension was recently placed on a calcium channel blocker and presents to the office complaining of swollen ankles. On examination, he weighs 80 kg and has a blood pressure of 160/90 mm Hg and 1+ pitting edema over his ankles. His blood urea is 30 mg/dl, and his creatinine is 1.3 mg/dl. His serum albumin is 3.8 mg/dl, and his serum cholesterol is 307 mg/dl. His urinalysis shows 2+ protein and no blood. The protein–creatinine ratio in urine is 0.35. Does this patient have nephrotic syndrome? What is the likely cause of this patient's proteinuria?

CASE DISCUSSION

This patient has edema and hyperlipidemia but does not have hypoproteinemia or nephrotic-range proteinuria as assessed by his urine protein–creatinine ratio. This patient's long-standing hypertension has probably led to nephrosclerosis and low-grade proteinuria. This patient's edema is probably caused by his calcium channel blocker and resolves when he is switched to another antihypertensive medication.

SELECTED READING

Bernard DB, Salant DJ. Clinical approach to the patient with proteinuria and the nephrotic syndrome. In: Jacobson HR, Striker GE, Klahr S, eds. The principles and practice of nephrology. Philadelphia: BC Decker, 1991.

Cohen EP, Lemann J Jr. The role of the laboratory in evaluation of kidney function. Clin Chem 1991;37:785.

Hricik DE, Smith MC. Proteinuria and the nephrotic syndrome. Chicago: Year Book Medical Publishers, 1986.

Kanwar YS, Liu ZZ, Kashihara N, Wallner EI. Current status of the structural and functional basis of glomerular filtration and proteinuria. Semin Nephrol 1991;11:390.

Kelsch RC, Sedman AB. Nephrotic syndrome. Pediatr Rev 1983;14:30.

Keren DK. High resolution electrophoresis and immunofixation. Boston: Butterworths, 1987.

Lippincott's Pathophysiology Series: Renal Pathophysiology, edited by James A. Shayman. J. B. Lippincott Company, Philadelphia © 1995.

CHAPTER

6

Hematuria

William E. Smoyer

OBJECTIVES

By the end of this chapter the reader should be able to:

- Define microhematuria and macrohematuria.
- Describe the important questions in the history of a patient with hematuria.
- Describe the important physical examination findings in a patient with hematuria.
- Describe the important laboratory findings in a patient with hematuria.
- Outline an approach to the patient with hematuria.
- Describe the various causes of hematuria and of discolored urine in the absence of hematuria.
- Define glomerulonephritis.
- Describe the major causes for glomerulonephritis and their general management principles.
- Describe the immunologic theories of the pathogenesis of the common forms of glomerulonephritis.

When a patient presents with blood in the urine, or hematuria, identification of the cause is essential in guiding the physician to choose what therapy, if any, is indicated. The goal of this chapter is to help the reader develop a logical approach to the diagnosis and treatment of patient with hematuria. Important aspects of the patient history, physical examination, and laboratory evaluation relevant to the evaluation of hematuria are emphasized. The major causes for hematuria, as well as glomerulonephritis, are to be discussed. Cases are presented that illustrate the approach to patients with hematuria, with emphasis on the clinical presentation, diagnosis, pathogenesis, and management of common forms of glomerulonephritis.

DEFINITIONS

It is not unusual to find one or two red blood cells in the urine of most people. The number of urinary red blood cells that distinguishes normal excretion from disease states, however, has not been precisely defined. In practice, most physicians consider more than four red blood cells per high power microscope field in fresh, spun urine to be abnormal. This value correlates with approximately two to eight red blood cells/mm^3 in fresh, unspun urine and an approximate red blood cell excretion rate of 10,000 cells/hour.

Hematuria may be either microscopic (i.e., *microhematuria*) or macroscopic (i.e., *macrohematuria* or *gross hematuria*). Macroscopic hematuria is visible to the naked eye. Most often, the urine is red to brown in color, but it may be described as tea-, rust-, or cola-colored. In contrast, microscopic hematuria can be detected only by urine examination under a microscope or by urine dipstick. The urine appears clear and yellow to the unaided eye.

In some situations, urine may be discolored in the absence of true hematuria. Microscopic examination of the urine will confirm the absence of red blood cells. Common causes for discolored urine in the absence of red cells include heme pigments (i.e., hemoglobin and myoglobin), porphyrins, and azo dyes, which are usually present as a result of foods or drugs. With the exceptions of hemoglobinuria and myoglobinuria, the causes of discolored urine are all negative by dipstick evaluation. When a patient presents with discolored urine, the initial evaluation should always include a urine dipstick and microscopic analysis to determine if the patient truly has hematuria.

It is often useful to make a distinction between patients with hematuria only and those with hematuria associated with other laboratory or clinical findings. If isolated microscopic hematuria (otherwise normal history, examination, and urinalysis) alone is detected at initial evaluation, a repeat urine sample should be obtained in a few days or weeks before further evaluation is conducted. In one large study in children, repeat urine dipstick evaluations revealed that only one half of the subjects had hematuria that persisted on the second and third urine collections. Blood should be present in at least two of three urine specimens to confirm the diagnosis of isolated microscopic hematuria. In most situations, isolated hematuria is transient and not indicative of a disease state. The incidence of hematuria in the general public is approximately 1%, as defined by the presence of blood in at least two urine collections.

PATIENT HISTORY

A careful history is essential in determining the basis for hematuria. Frequently, a presumptive diagnosis can be made, but in almost all cases, the history helps to direct further evaluation. The important patient history issues helpful in the evaluation of hematuria are listed in Table 6-1. Several precipitating events may result in hematuria. A dietary history combined with absence of red cells on urinalysis might reveal a drug-, food-, or disease-related cause for discolored urine. A history of a sore throat or skin infection 1 to 3 weeks prior to the onset of hematuria, especially when hypertension or edema are present, is suggestive of postinfectious glomerulonephritis. In contrast, episodes of gross hematuria associated with concurrent upper respiratory tract infections is highly suggestive of IgA nephropathy. A history of blunt trauma may suggest the presence of kidney rupture or damage to the ureters or bladder. Vigorous exercise also can sometimes induce mild, transient hematuria.

The signs and symptoms associated with hematuria can help to localize its origin. Edema, hypertension, and oliguria are often seen with acute glomerulonephritis. In contrast, dysuria, urinary frequency, and flank pain are hallmarks of urinary tract infection. Other causes for dysuria include nephrolithiasis and hypercalciuria. The classic malar rash of systemic lupus erythematosus or the petechial or purpuric lower-extremity rash seen with Henoch-Schönlein purpura are almost diagnostic of themselves.

Several preexisting conditions and medications may be responsible for hematuria. Patients with congenital heart disease or chronic lung disease often have a history of prolonged use of loop diuretics (usually furosemide), which predisposes them to the development of hypercalciuria and subsequent hematuria. Patients being treated with anticoagulants are also at risk for hematuria. Cyclophosphamide therapy can induce hemorrhagic cystitis in patients who are not adequately hydrated. Several medications, including antibiotics, nonsteroidal anti-inflammatory agents, and loop diuretics can cause tubulointerstitial nephritis, in which nonoliguric acute renal failure may be accompanied by fever, rash, and sometimes pyuria or hematuria. Neoplasms anywhere in the urinary tract, as well as their therapies, including chemotherapy, surgery, and radiation, may result in hematuria. Because of their frequent association with hematuria, cystic kidney disease, nephrolithiasis, sickle cell disease or trait, and systemic lupus erythematosus should also be excluded. Neonatal complications such as renal venous or arterial thrombosis may also present with hematuria.

A thorough family history may reveal a hereditary cause for hematuria. The presence of any family members with renal failure or a history of renal transplantation should alert the physician to the possibility of several heritable diseases. A history of hematuria, deafness, and renal failure in male relatives strongly suggests Alport's syndrome, whereas a history of older relatives on dialysis and family members having had cerebral vascular accidents is suspicious for polycystic kidney disease. Sickle cell disease or trait in a patient's family warrants screening for this disease, because either can be responsible for hematuria. Fabry's disease and nail–patella syndrome are rare inherited causes for hematuria. Familial associations exist also for nephrolithiasis, IgA nephropathy, and systemic lupus erythematosus.

PHYSICAL EXAMINATION

Careful physical examination, although not usually diagnostic, can be of significant help in directing further evaluation of the patient with hematuria (Table 6-2). Hypertension and edema in the presence of hematuria comprise the *nephritic syndrome,* which is classic for glomerulonephritis. These patients sometimes also

TABLE 6-1. *PATIENT HISTORY IN THE EVALUATION OF HEMATURIA*

Precipitating events
    Diet
    Respiratory infections
    Skin infections
    Trauma
    Vigorous exercise
Associated signs and symptoms
    Arthralgia
    Dysuria
    Edema
    Flank or back pain
    Oliguria or anuria
    Polyuria
    Rash
    Urinary urgency or frequency
Past history
    Congenital heart disease
    Cystic kidney disease
    Diabetes
    Malignancy
    Medications
        Antibiotics
        Anticoagulants (e.g., Coumadin, heparin)
        Cyclophosphamide
        Loop diuretics
        Nonsteroidal antiinflammatory agents
    Neonatal complications
    Nephrolithiasis
    Sickle cell disease or trait
    Systemic lupus erythematosus
Family history
    Chronic renal failure or dialysis
    Cystic kidney disease
    Deafness
    Hematuria
    Nephrolithiasis
    Sickle cell disease or trait
    Systemic lupus erythematosus

TABLE 6-2. *PHYSICAL EXAMINATION FINDINGS IN THE EVALUATION OF HEMATURIA*

Abdominal bruit

Abdominal mass or masses

Arthritis

Ascites

Congestive heart failure (e.g., tachycardia, tachypnea, rales)

Edema (e.g., periorbital, scrotal, pedal)

Flank tenderness

Hypertension

Pharyngeal erythema or exudate

Rashes (e.g., petechial, purpuric, impetiginous, malar)

Urethral trauma, stenosis, or discharge

have signs of congestive heart failure with tachycardia, gallop, tachypnea, and rales. Generalized edema, with or without ascites, associated with massive proteinuria and less frequently hematuria, can be seen with nephrotic syndrome resulting from several glomerular lesions. An erythematous pharynx or other signs of upper respiratory infection during an episode of gross hematuria is suggestive of IgA nephropathy. A resolving sore throat or impetiginous skin lesion in the same setting, however, is more consistent with a postinfectious (i.e., poststreptococcal) glomerulonephritis. Arthritis and a malar or butterfly rash on the face with hematuria, proteinuria, and sometimes renal insufficiency can be seen in patients with systemic lupus erythematosus. A purpuric or petechial rash over the lower extremities or buttocks in association with abdominal pain, arthralgia, and hematuria or proteinuria is highly suggestive of Henoch-Schönlein purpura. Flank tenderness may be found in association with upper urinary tract infection, nephrolithiasis, or urinary tract obstruction. Identification of an abdominal mass on palpation may indicate the presence of urinary tract obstruction, malignancy, or polycystic kidney disease. An abdominal bruit in the presence of hypertension should induce suspicion of renal vascular disease, in which hematuria may be seen as a manifestation of end-organ damage. Urethral trauma, stenosis, or infection, which is suggested by the presence of a discharge, are also causes for hematuria.

LABORATORY STUDIES

The initial laboratory investigation of any patient with suspected hematuria should include dipstick analysis of the urine for specific gravity, pH, blood, and protein, as well as microscopic evaluation for the presence of cellular elements and casts. The urine reagent strips used to screen for hematuria (e.g., Chemstrip, Multistix, Labstix) are impregnated with orthotolidine peroxide and enhanced with 6-methoxyquinolone, resulting in a blue color change in the presence of either hemoglobin or myoglobin. False-positive tests occur rarely in urine infected with bacteria producing large amounts of peroxidase. False-negative results also occur rarely in the presence of high concentrations of ascorbic acid. A positive result correlates approximately with more than 2 red blood cells per high power field in a fresh, spun urine sample. Persistent positive urine dipstick results in the presence of more than 5 red blood cells per high power field confirms the presence of abnormal hematuria.

After hematuria has been confirmed, determination of whether the bleeding is coming from the upper urinary tract (kidneys) or lower urinary tract (renal pelvis, ureters, bladder, urethra) can significantly narrow the diagnostic possibilities. Upper urinary tract bleeding generally results in brown or tea-colored urine, because the acidic urine converts the hemoglobin to hematin, which produces a brown color. Bright red blood is more suggestive of lower urinary tract bleeding. The presence of proteinuria also helps to localize the source of bleeding to the glomerulus, where the protein is presumably leaking across damaged glomerular basement membranes. Proteinuria of 1+ or more on dipstick should be quantitated with a 24-hour urine collection. Values greater than 10 mg/M^2/hour are abnormal and require further evaluation. Identification of red cell casts in the urine are highly suggestive of a glomerular cause and should prompt a more extensive evaluation for causes of glomerulonephritis (Fig. 6-1A). Gross hematuria originating in the lower urinary tract rarely results in significant proteinuria. The presence of blood clots or blood noted only at the beginning or end of urination also implies a lower urinary tract cause.

Analysis of red blood cell morphology also can sometimes help to identify the source of bleeding (Fig. 6-1B). Dysmorphic red blood cells are thought to result from damage to their cell membranes as they pass through the glomerular basement membrane. In contrast, normally shaped cells suggest a more distal cause for hematuria. Unfortunately, this analysis is best performed using a phase contrast microscope, which is not available in most laboratories. In addition, there can be a significant degree of overlap between causes for dysmorphic and normally shaped cells, resulting in one author's suggestion that upper urinary tract bleeding be diagnosed only if more than 75% of red blood cells are dysmorphic and lower urinary tract disease only if less than 17% of red blood cells are abnormally shaped.

The presence of an abnormal number (5 white blood cells/high power field) of white blood cells in the urine (i.e., pyuria) suggests urinary tract inflammation (Fig. 6-2). This condition may be noted in glomerulonephritis, tubulointerstitial nephritis, or urinary tract infection. Although a urine culture is not routinely necessary in the evaluation of hematuria, a culture should be obtained in the presence of pyuria, especially if bacteria are seen under the microscope or if the dipstick is positive for leukocyte esterase and nitrite. White blood cell casts also may be seen in cases of pyelonephritis. A repeat urinalysis following treatment of any urinary tract infection allows the exclusion of persistent hematuria. Tubulointerstitial nephritis may be suggested by drug history, coexistence of proteinuria, or findings of fever, arthralgias, or rash.

In patients who present with isolated hematuria without an obvious cause, several studies may help identify the cause. A spot urine calcium–creatinine ratio greater than 0.2 is suggestive of hypercalciuria and warrants a 24-hour urine collection for actual quantitation of daily calcium excretion. Urinalyses on other family members may help identify familial causes such as benign familial hematuria or hereditary nephritis. A renal ultrasound may be used to exclude the possibilities of urinary tract obstruction, polycystic kidneys, nephrolithiasis, and malignancy.

If glomerulonephritis is suspected, serum studies can be very helpful in identifying its cause. Routine studies include a complete blood count (CBC), elec-

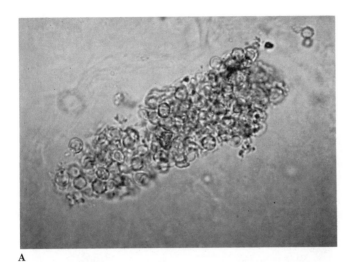

A

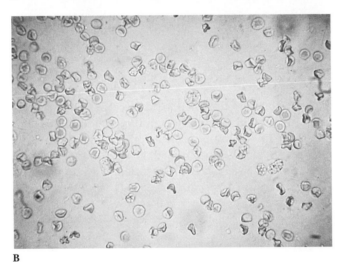

B

Figure 6-1. (A) Red blood cell cast. (B) Dysmorphic red blood cells. (Picture reproduced with permission from Haber MH. Urine casts, their microscopy and clinical significance. Chicago: American Society of Clinical Pathologists, 1976.)

trolytes, blood urea nitrogen (BUN), creatinine, C3 complement, C4 complement, and antinuclear antibody (ANA). If edema or nephrotic-range proteinuria (>40 mg/M^2/hour) is present, serum albumin and cholesterol should also be tested to document the presence or absence of the nephrotic syndrome. A depressed C3 complement level may be seen with membranoproliferative glomerulonephritis, lupus nephritis, poststreptococcal glomerulonephritis, or other causes of postinfectious glomerulonephritis.

Poststreptococcal nephritis can be confirmed by a history of sore throat or skin infection and a positive Streptozyme test, which detects antibodies against any of five extracellular products of streptococci. Lupus nephritis is most often accompanied by a suggestive history and positive ANA, although further serology, such as antibodies to double-stranded DNA, may be needed for confirmation. Hepatitis B serology may detect a postinfectious glomerulonephritis caused by this virus. In black patients, a sickle cell preparation or hemoglobin electrophoresis could un-

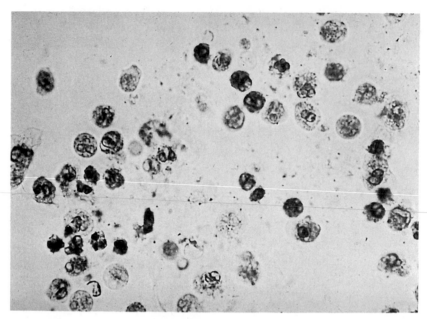

Figure 6-2. White blood cells on urinalysis.

cover the presence of sickle disease or trait. In patients with accompanying respiratory- or sinus-related complaints, a serum antineutrophil cytoplasmic antibody (ANCA) titer may identify a form of rapidly progressive glomerulonephritis referred to as pauci-immune to describe the absence of glomerular immune deposits on renal biopsy. If the serum creatinine, adjusted for the patient's age, is abnormally elevated in the setting of presumed glomerulonephritis, the patient should be referred to a nephrologist for consideration of a renal biopsy.

DIAGNOSTIC APPROACH

An extensive but incomplete list of the causes of hematuria arising from each segment of the urinary tract is displayed in Table 6-3. Using the previously described patient history, physical examination, and laboratory findings commonly associated with hematuria, a series of cases are provided to outline a diagnostic approach to the patient presenting with hematuria. Emphasis is placed on the diagnosis, pathogenesis, and general management principles of glomerulonephritis.

CASE 1

A 17-year-old black boy presents to the office with a complaint of new-onset dark brown urine this morning. He has no dysuria or flank pain, but noted mild swelling around his eyes this morning. Further questioning reveals only a vague history of skin lesions on his lower legs 2 to 3 weeks ago and sickle cell trait in two cousins. Physical examination reveals a blood pressure of 154/95 mm Hg, mild periorbital and pedal edema, and scattered healing erythematous skin lesions on the lower legs. Urinalysis reveals 3+ blood, 2+ protein, and a single red cell cast. Serum electrolytes are normal, the BUN is 28 mg/dl and the creatinine is 1.4 mg/dl.

TABLE 6-3. *CAUSES OF HEMATURIA*

Renal
  Glomerular
    Proliferative
      Essential mixed cryoglobulinemia
      Goodpasture's syndrome
      Henoch–Schönlein nephritis
      IgA nephropathy
      Lupus glomerulonephritis
      Membranoproliferative glomerulonephritis
      Postinfectious glomerulonephritis
      Rapidly progressive glomerulonephritis
    Nonproliferative
      Benign familial hematuria
      Fabry's disease
      Focal Glomerulosclerosis, global and segmental
      Hereditary nephritis
      Minimal–change nephrotic syndrome
      Membranous nephropathy
      Nail–patella syndrome
      Nephrosclerosis (e.g., diabetic, hypertensive)
      Vasculitic damage (i.e., microangiopathy)
  Nonglomerular
    Developmental
      Medullary sponge kidney
      Polycystic kidney disease, autosomal dominant and recessive
      Simple cysts
    Tubulointerstitial nephropathy
      Acute tubular necrosis
      Allergic vasculitis
      Drug-induced (e.g., antibiotics, nonsteroidal antiinflammatory agents)
      Infectious (e.g., pyelonephritis)
      Metabolic (e.g., nephrocalcinosis, oxalate, uric acid)
    Tumors
      Angiomyolipoma (i.e., tuberous sclerosis)
      Renal cell carcinoma
      Wilm's tumor

(continued)

TABLE 6-3. *CAUSES OF HEMATURIA (CONTINUED)*

Vascular
  Analgesic abuse
  Malformations (e.g., aneurysm, arteriovenous fistula, hemangioma)
  Renal venous or arterial thrombosis
  Sickle cell nephropathy

Pelvic and ureteral
  Infection
  Obstruction
  Trauma
  Tumor (i.e., transitional cell carcinoma)
  Urolithiasis
  Vascular malformations

Vesical
  Drugs (e.g., cyclophosphamide)
  Infection or inflammation
  Obstruction
  Stones
  Trauma
  Tumors (transitional cell carcinoma)
  Vascular malformations

Urethral
  Infection or inflammation
  Squamous cell carcinoma
  Trauma

Other
  Anticoagulants (e.g., heparin, Coumadin)
  Endometriosis
  Exercise-induced hematuria
  Factitious
  Fabry's disease
  Hypercalciuria
  Juvenile rheumatoid arthritis
  Loin–pain hematuria syndrome
  Nail–patella syndrome
  Prostate or epididymal infection
  Prostatic hypertrophy or adenocarcinoma

CASE DISCUSSION

The clinical features of hematuria, proteinuria, azotemia, hypertension, and edema in this patient characterize the *nephritic syndrome* and are the hallmarks of acute glomerulonephritis. The term glomerulonephritis describes a group of renal diseases in which the major injury takes place in the glomeruli, rather than in the tubules, vessels, or interstitium of the kidney. Glomerulonephritis is confirmed by the finding of even a single red blood cell cast in the urine. In the acute forms of glomerulonephritis, there is typically an abrupt onset of signs and symptoms, and although diagnosis does not require all of these signs, edema and hematuria occur most commonly. The most common forms of acute glomerulonephritis include IgA nephropathy (i.e., Berger's Disease), poststreptococcal glomerulonephritis, lupus nephritis, and membranoproliferative glomerulonephritis. The history of a skin infection 2 to 3 weeks prior to the onset of gross hematuria and the presence of healing skin lesions (presumably impetiginous) on the legs on examination make poststreptococcal glomerulonephritis the most likely diagnosis in this patient.

Poststreptococcal glomerulonephritis usually occurs 1 to 3 weeks following a throat or skin (impetigo) infection with specific strains of group A β-hemolytic streptococci. It occurs more commonly in children than adults. Although proteinuria and microscopic hematuria are present in all patients, approximately 30% to 65% of children and 30% of adults admitted to the hospital present with gross hematuria. Edema, hypertension, or both are present in approximately three fourths of patients and are primarily the result of salt and water retention caused by a reduced glomerular filtration rate. The diagnosis is usually confirmed by the history, examination findings, abnormal serum streptozyme test (positive in 80% to 95% of patients), and the presence of a low serum C3 complement level, which is depressed in 90% of patients in the first weeks of illness. Clinical identification of this disease is particularly important, because spontaneous recovery is usually seen, and renal biopsy is not indicated.

When the clinical diagnosis of poststreptococcal glomerulonephritis is in doubt, a renal biopsy may be helpful. The disease is characterized histologically by glomerular hypercellularity caused by proliferation of mesangial and endothelial cells, and infiltration of the glomeruli by immune cells, including neutrophils and macrophages. This infiltration results in narrowing or even closure of the capillary lumens and is the etiology of the decreased glomerular filtration rate (Fig. 6-3).

The immunologic mechanism involved in the pathogenesis of poststreptococcal glomerulonephritis is unknown. One suggestion is that nephritogenic (i.e., disease-producing) streptococci may contain a unique cationic antigen that allows binding to the negatively charged glomerular basement membrane. Immune recognition of the deposits by antistreptococcal antibodies may then activate complement and result in the formation of the classic subepithelial immune deposits (i.e., humps) seen in renal biopsy specimens of these patients. Another theory proposes that nephritogenic streptococci release an enzyme, neuraminidase, that is capable of both making endogenous IgG antigenic and increasing its affinity for the glomerulus. Resultant anti-IgG–IgG immune complexes could then be formed in the kidney and induce an inflammatory response.

Therapy for poststreptococcal glomerulonephritis is generally supportive.

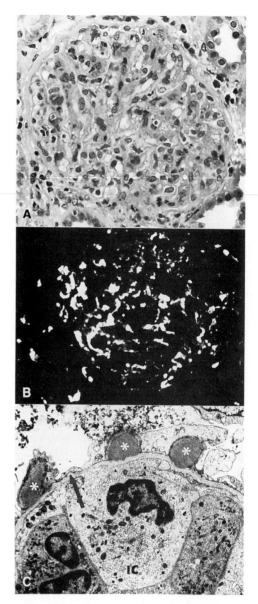

Figure 6-3. Renal biopsy findings of acute post-streptococcal glomerulonephritis. (**A**) Prominent polymorphonuclear leukocytes in a swollen glomerular tuft. (**B**) Granular deposits of IgG in the mesangial region and glomerular basement membrane. (**C**) Electron micrograph (× 5400) showing epimembranous deposits (*asterisks*) along the glomerular basement membrane (*arrows*). (From Knutson DW, Abt AB. Immune-mediated glomerulopathies. In: Kelley WN, ed. Textbook of internal medicine. 2nd ed. Philadelphia: JB Lippincott, 1992:705.)

The use of loop diuretics often helps remove the excess fluid and lower blood pressure in patients who are edematous or hypertensive. Good control of blood pressure with antihypertensives is important to prevent the occurrence of hypertensive encephalopathy. In patients who were previously normotensive, a sudden rise in blood pressure to even moderate levels can precipitate the onset of headache, restlessness, nausea, vomiting, confusion, or focal neurologic abnormalities. These abnormalities usually resolve in 1 to 2 days with appropriate management.

The vast majority of patients with poststreptococcal glomerulonephritis recover completely, and even in those patients who present with advanced acute renal failure, most will experience onset of diuresis within 1 week, with normalization of renal function within 3 to 4 weeks. Hematuria may persist for 6 weeks, and proteinuria may last for many months. Despite recovery from the acute episode, some patients develop hypertension, proteinuria, or renal insufficiency as long as 10 to 40 years later, most likely as a result of irreversible damage during the acute illness. Less than 2% of patients progress to end-stage renal disease or die, and children have an even better prognosis than adults.

CASE 2

A 32-year-old Caucasian woman is referred for evaluation of presumed hematuria based on three urine dipstick evaluations over the last 2 months which revealed 2+ blood and 2+ protein. The referring physician reports she is asymptomatic and has a normal physical examination and blood pressure, and the family history is negative for hematuria, hearing deficits, or renal disease. How would you approach the evaluation of hematuria in this patient?

CASE DISCUSSION

Initial evaluation of any patient with suspected hematuria should include a careful history. Care should be taken to inquire about any abnormal findings on previous urinalyses, because this may help identify the time of onset of hematuria. Inquiry about associated signs and symptoms, past and family history, and for patients with gross hematuria, precipitating events (see Table 6-1) can greatly narrow the differential diagnosis. On questioning, this patient was able to recall a transient episode of brown urine several months ago which was painless and lasted 1 day. She had forgotten about it because she was menstruating at the time and had a cold.

A urinalysis should always be performed to confirm the presence of red blood cells and to look for proteinuria, pyuria, and casts. In this patient, urinalysis revealed 2+ protein, 2+ blood, 10 to 15 red blood cells/high power field, 3 to 5 white blood cells/high power field, and 1 red cell cast. A 24-hour urine collection revealed 1 g of protein. Distinguishing upper urinary tract from lower urinary tract causes for hematuria is one of the most helpful ways to narrow the diagnostic possibilities. The presence of proteinuria and a red cell cast localize the hematuria to the upper urinary tract and confirm the diagnosis of glomerulonephritis.

At this point, serum studies can help to exclude causes of glomerulonephritis such as lupus nephritis, membranoproliferative glomerulonephritis, and poststreptococcal glomerulonephritis, as well as identify any renal insufficiency. Appropriate tests include CBC, electrolytes, BUN, creatinine, serum ANA, and C3/C4. In this patient, notable findings include normal electrolytes, BUN, creatinine, and complement levels, and negative ANA. A urine calcium–creatinine ratio is normal at 0.1 (normal, <0.2). Renal ultrasonography shows 2 kidneys of normal size and echo texture, with no evidence for stones, obstruction, or malignancy.

This woman appears to have glomerulonephritis characterized by persistent microhematuria, an episode of probable painless, gross hematuria associated with a respiratory infection, and normal renal function, without any obvious cause after initial evaluation. The temporal association of gross hematuria with a respiratory infection in the setting of persistent microhematuria is often seen in patients with IgA nephropathy, however, and makes this the most likely of the remaining possibilities. To establish a diagnosis in this case, a renal biopsy is necessary. The biopsy is performed and the diagnosis of IgA nephropathy confirmed.

IgA nephropathy is probably the most common cause of glomerulonephritis in the world. Patients usually present either with asymptomatic microscopic hematuria or with episodes of gross hematuria. When present, the episodes often occur 1 to 3 days after an upper respiratory infection, or less commonly, after gastroenteritis. The gross hematuria generally lasts only a few days, but microscopic hematuria often persists. In more severe cases, patients can present with nephrotic syndrome, rental insufficiency, or both.

Renal biopsy is required to confirm the diagnosis of IgA nephropathy, which is characterized by immunofluorescent detection of IgA (as well as C3, IgG, and IgM) in the mesangium. Light microscopy usually reveals variable increases in mesangial cellularity and matrix in the majority of glomeruli, and is less specific (Fig. 6-4).

The etiology of IgA nephropathy is most often idiopathic, but several experimental observations and clinical reports, in addition to its association with various intestinal and pulmonary diseases, have led to suggestions of a variety of pathogenic mechanisms. It is generally agreed that IgA nephropathy is an immune complex glomerulonephritis caused by deposition of IgA immune complexes in the glomerular mesangium. Although the antigen (or antigens) to which the IgA

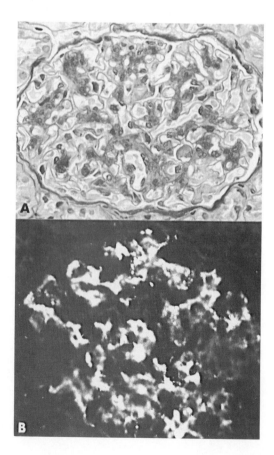

Figure 6-4. IgA nephropathy. (**A**) Mesangial proliferation with normal peripheral capillary basement membranes. (**B**) Mesangial staining of antihuman IgA. (From Knutson DW, Abt AB. Immune-mediated glomerulopathies. In: Kelley WN, ed. Textbook of internal medicine. 2nd ed. Philadelphia: JB Lippincott, 1992:711.)

binds in the circulation has not been identified, most patients appear to have a defect in the regulation of IgA and may have an exaggerated mucosal IgA response to environmental antigens (e.g., food-related, viral, bacterial). Support for this theory has come from reports of elevated serum IgA levels and circulating IgA-containing immune complexes that parallel disease activity, and IgA deposition in normal skin following an upper respiratory infection in many patients. Increased numbers of circulating IgA-specific B and T cells have also been noted in some patients following upper respiratory infection. It has also been suggested that various combinations of three pathogenetic factors may be responsible for the manifestations this disease, including increased mucosal entry of environmental antigens and stimulation of an IgA response, impaired IgA immune response resulting in the production of abnormal macromolecular IgA, and impaired or saturated clearance of the macromolecular IgA. Despite these suggestions, there is evidence that chronic deposition of either normal or abnormal IgA in the glomerular mesangium alone is not sufficient to produce glomerular injury. Both human and animal studies have documented mesangial IgA deposition in the absence of any renal disease.

No specific therapy has been shown to be effective in altering the course of IgA nephropathy. Multiple reports suggest that neither prednisone nor cytotoxic agents are helpful, except in a minority of patients who present with the nephrotic syndrome and minimal glomerular abnormalities on biopsy. These patients often behave clinically in a manner similar to patients with minimal-change nephrotic syndrome. Other attempted therapies have included phenytoin or danazol to alter the abnormal immune response, plasma exchange to remove circulating immune complexes, and prophylactic antibiotics or tonsillectomy to prevent potential entry of infectious agents. Although previously thought to be a relatively benign disease, recent studies have shown that 20% to 30% of adults will develop chronic renal failure 20 years after initial diagnosis, whereas the incidence in children has been reported to be 11% at 15 years from diagnosis.

CASE 3

A 27-year-old Caucasian woman presents with a 3-week history of feeling tired. On questioning, she points out that she has also had mild arthralgias in her wrists and hands since last week. The only other pertinent patient history finding is a strong family history of hypertension. Pertinent examination findings include a blood pressure of 148/97 mm Hg and mild swelling and erythema of the wrists and phalangeal joints. Urinalysis reveals 1+ blood, 2+ protein, 5 to 10 red blood cells/high power field, 3 to 5 white blood cells/high power field, and 1 to 3 granular casts. Renal function and electrolytes are normal. What diagnoses are most compatible with these findings, and what tests should be ordered at this point?

CASE DISCUSSION

This patient presents with microhematuria, proteinuria, and hypertension. Unlike the previous case, however, she does not have the edema and azotemia seen in the classic presentation for acute glomerulonephritis. The important clues here are the history of tiredness and the nonrenal findings of arthralgias and arthritis. These findings should raise suspicion for diagnoses such as lupus nephritis or Henoch-Schönlein nephritis, although these findings can be seen with tubulointerstitial nephritis as well.

Because the presence of both hematuria and proteinuria suggests an upper urinary tract cause for the hematuria, appropriate tests include routine laboratory studies to exclude the various causes of glomerulonephritis: CBC, electrolytes, BUN, creatinine, ANA, C3/C4, and a 24-hour urine collection for protein (and creatinine, to document adequacy of the collection). The abnormal findings in this patient are a 24-hour urine protein excretion of 820 mg (normal, <150 mg/24 hours), C3 level of 28 mg/dl (normal, 80–231 mg/dl), and a positive ANA at 1:160 with a speckled pattern. These results all point toward systemic lupus erythematosus as the primary disease process. This is confirmed by documentation of circulating antibodies to native (i.e., double-stranded) DNA.

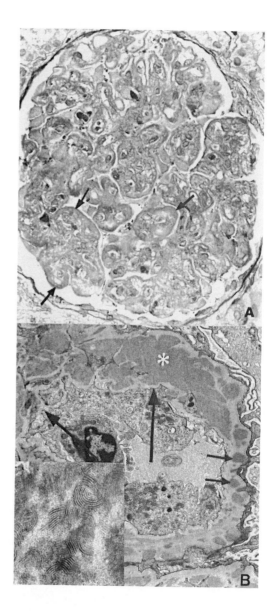

Figure 6-5. Diffuse proliferative glomerulonephritis in systemic lupus erythematosus. (**A**) Cellular proliferation and thickened glomerular basement membranes (*arrows*). (**B**) Electron micrograph (× 5200) showing subendothelial deposits (*asterisk*) and intramembranous deposits (*arrows*). *Inset:* "Fingerprint" pattern within the deposits often seen with lupus glomerulonephritis. (From Knutson DW, Abt AB. Immune-mediated glomerulopathies. In: Kelley WN, ed. Textbook of internal medicine. 2nd ed. Philadelphia: JB Lippincott, 1992:714.)

Systemic lupus erythematosus has a strong predilection for females, who comprise 90% of all cases. The typical presentation is with systemic complaints such as fatigue, malar rash, pleuritis, and arthralgias. Renal involvement has been noted in approximately one half of patients at the time of diagnosis, and ultimately in greater than three fourths of patients.

In the majority of patients with suspected systemic lupus, a renal biopsy is not necessary to confirm the diagnosis. If there is evidence of renal involvement, however, a renal biopsy is indicated to assess the degree of renal disease and guide institution of appropriate therapy. Four separate forms of glomerular involvement have been described in systemic lupus: mesangial, focal proliferative, diffuse proliferative, and membranous. Diffuse proliferative glomerulonephritis is the most common type and is seen in 40% to 60% of biopsy specimens. This lesion is characterized by diffuse proliferative and necrotizing glomerular lesions, with diffuse granular immunofluorescent staining for IgG, IgM, C3, C4, and sometimes IgA.

The pathogenesis of systemic lupus revolves around the formation of autoantibodies. The immunologic mechanism for renal involvement in disease is thought to be glomerular deposition of DNA–αDNA immune complexes, with subsequent complement activation and recruitment of inflammatory cells. Immune complexes are initially deposited in the mesangium (leading to mesangial lupus), but if the number of complexes deposited overwhelms the ability of the mesangium to clear them, the deposits spread to the nearby subendothelial spaces, resulting in focal or diffuse proliferative lupus nephritis. In contrast to the glomerular deposition of preformed immune complexes, membranous lupus nephritis is thought to result from the formation of immune complexes across the glomerular basement membrane in the subepithelial spaces (Fig. 6-5).

Therapy for lupus nephritis varies with the type of glomerular lesion. Diffuse proliferative disease requires treatment with either prednisone alone in mild cases or with combinations of steroids and cyclophosphamide for more severe disease. The other three types of lesions do not require any specific therapy, but renal function and urinalyses must be followed closely, because transformation to diffuse proliferative nephritis with progressive renal insufficiency can occur.

SUMMARY

Hematuria may originate from several areas of the urinary tract. With a careful patient history, including past and family histories and documentation of any associated signs and symptoms, the diagnostic possibilities can be greatly narrowed. The ability to distinguish between an upper or lower urinary tract cause can also help guide the evaluation of hematuria. In some patients with isolated microscopic hematuria, the etiology may remain uncertain after initial evaluation, yet further studies may not be warranted. In contrast, a cause almost always can and should be determined for patients presenting with gross hematuria.

SELECTED READING

Boineau FG, Lewy JE. Evaluation of hematuria in children and adolescents. Pediatr Rev 1989;11:101.

Kelley WN, ed. Essentials of internal medicine. Philadelphia: JB Lippincott, 1994: Chapters 47 and 50.

Rose DB, Black RM. Manual of clinical problems in nephrology. Boston: Little, Brown and Company, 1988.

Lippincott's Pathophysiology Series: Renal Pathophysiology, edited by James A. Shayman. J. B. Lippincott Company, Philadelphia © 1995.

CHAPTER

7

Acute Renal Failure

H. David Humes

OBJECTIVES

By the end of this chapter the reader should be able to:

- Understand the three pathophysiologic classifications of acute renal failure.
- Calculate the fractional excretion of sodium (FE_{Na}) and apply this value in the differential diagnosis of prerenal versus intrarenal acute renal failure.
- Know the common etiologies of prerenal acute renal failure.
- Understand the causes and histologic patterns associated with acute tubular necrosis.
- Understand the distinction between intrarenal and extrarenal obstruction as a cause of acute renal failure.

Acute rental failure is a common clinical syndrome. It is defined as an abrupt decline in renal function. The clinical manifestations of this disorder arise from the decline in glomerular filtration rate (GFR) and the inability of the kidney to excrete the toxic wastes produced by the body. It is recognized clinically by rising levels of blood urea nitrogen (BUN) and creatinine and usually a reduced urine output, and it may present dramatically, with a patient progressing from normal renal function to uremia within 1 week. Most forms of acute renal failure are reversible processes; therefore, correct diagnosis and management of this disorder are critical to allow time for improvement of renal function to occur.

The distinction between acute, subacute, and chronic renal failure is somewhat arbitrary. Most physicians accept the definition of acute renal failure as a rise in plasma creatinine of 0.5 mg/dl/day and a rise in BUN of 10 mg/dl/day over several days. Using these criteria, the syndrome can best be categorized into *prerenal (i.e., functional)*, *intrarenal (i.e., structural)*, and *postrenal (i.e., obstructive) causes*.

PRERENAL ACUTE RENAL FAILURE

Prerenal acute renal failure, or prerenal azotemia, results from a persistent, significant decline in renal blood flow (RBF). Because the rate of glomerular filtration is highly dependent on RBF, a decline in RBF results in a decrease in GFR and an increase in levels of BUN and serum creatinine. Usually, this decline in renal perfusion is a component of a generalized condition involving poor tissue perfusion, such as hypotension, dehydration, or the edematous state of congestive heart failure, cirrhosis, or the nephrotic syndrome (Table 7-1).

ETIOLOGY

A decline in absolute or relative effective arterial blood volume results in a decrease in perfusion of vital organs and a fall in mean arterial pressure. Both central and peripheral baroreceptors are activated to initiate compensatory mechanisms, including increases in cardiac contractility and venous and arteriolar vasoconstriction, to improve the perfusion of vital organs and maintain blood pressure. A variety of vasoactive substances are released locally and systemically to promote arteriolar contraction, primarily in the renal, splanchnic, and musculocutaneous circulatory beds. At the renal level, sympathetic amines and angiotensin II are important hormones released locally to induce this response. Substantial declines in RBF and thus in GFR result in these conditions.

TABLE 7-1. *COMMON CAUSES OF PRERENAL ACUTE RENAL FAILURE*

Hypotension
Volume depletion
   Absolute
   Relative
Edema-forming states

Besides producing a fall in RBF, *hypotension* is associated with a lowering of the hydrostatic pressure in the glomerular capillary network. Because the hydrostatic pressure in the glomerulus is the major driving force for glomerular filtration, GFR consequently falls. Thus, a decline in systemic blood pressure results both in a decrease in RBF and a lowering of glomerular capillary hydrostatic pressure, both of which lead to a decline in GFR (Fig. 7-1).

Absolute *volume depletion* secondary to sodium loss (see Chap. 2) can also lead to prerenal azotemia. The decline in extracellular volume results in absolute reductions in intravascular volume, cardiac output, RBF, and GFR. Prerenal acute renal failure can also occur in the *edematous disorders*. In congestive heart failure, prerenal azotemia can occur from either a reduction in cardiac output secondary to intrinsic cardiac processes and subsequent declines in RBF, or more commonly, from a further reduction in cardiac output from the use of diuretics to relieve pulmonary congestion and peripheral edema. Similar processes may produce renal impairment in other edematous disorders. In the nephrotic syndrome, the hypoalbuminemia results in a fall in plasma oncotic pressure and movement of fluid from

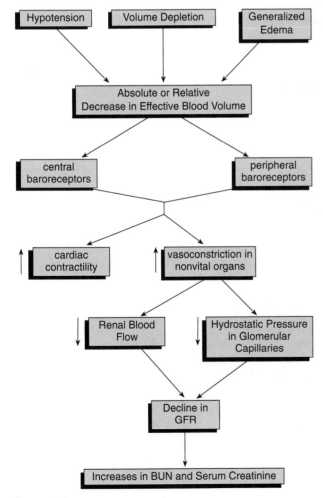

Figure 7-1.

the intravascular volume to the interstitial space. In cirrhosis of the liver, elevated portal venous pressure results in sequestration of volume in the mesenteric vascular system and fluid loss into the peritoneal cavity. Both disease states are thereby associated with declines in effective circulating volume and the potential to develop prerenal azotemia as a result of declines in RBF.

CASE 1

A 68-year-old man with biventricular heart failure from hypertension and atherosclerotic vascular disease is admitted to the hospital because of increasing shortness of breath, orthopnea, and paroxysmal nocturnal dyspnea over the past 10 days. The patient acknowledges a 5-kg weight gain and increasing ankle swelling over the previous week. He is on digoxin, 0.25 mg daily, and furosemide, 80 mg once daily. On physical examination, the patient has wet rales bilaterally. Laboratory values are as follows: serum Na, 133 mEq/L; serum creatinine, 1.8 mg/dl; and BUN, 36 mg/dl.

The patient is placed on bed rest, and his diuretic regimen is changed to furosemide, 120 mg twice daily, and metolazone, 5 mg once daily. Over the subsequent 3 days, the patient loses 8 kg, with marked clinical improvement. During this period, the patient's BUN rises from 36 to 60 mg/dl, and his serum creatinine rises from 1.8 to 2.5 mg/dl.

CASE DISCUSSION

This patient presents with signs and symptoms of both left and right ventricular failure. Consequently, reduced tissue perfusion develops, and cardiac output is maintained at the expense of high ventricular filling pressures, which cause both pulmonary and peripheral edema. The mildly elevated BUN and serum creatinine and the BUN–serum creatinine ratio of 20:1 reflect reduced renal perfusion. Diuretic therapy is increased and leads to a decline in ventricular filling pressures and partial elimination of edema fluid. Further reduction in tissue perfusion, as reflected by the further rise in BUN, serum creatinine, and BUN–creatinine ratio, also occurs.

DIAGNOSIS

Acute renal failure on a prerenal hemodynamic basis initially must be distinguished from acute renal failure secondary to intrarenal or postrenal causes by obtaining a careful patient history, by careful physical examination, and by evaluating key laboratory tests. Important evaluative points for the diagnosis of acute renal failure resulting from intrarenal and postrenal causes are detailed later in this chapter. In patients with absolute volume depletion and dehydration, there may be a history of vomiting, diarrhea, or diuretic use. Physical examination may reveal poor skin turgor, orthostatic hypotension, and tachycardia. Conversely, patients with relative declines in effective arterial blood volume from congestive heart failure, nephrotic syndrome, or cirrhosis may have peripheral edema, ascites, or both.

Because functional prerenal disease occurs in a kidney that is not intrinsically diseased, the urinalysis usually is unremarkable except for the relatively nonspecific appearance of an increased number of hyaline and granular casts (Fig. 7-2). Chemical determinants of the urine, however, are extremely useful. The renal response to diminished perfusion is avid salt and water reabsorption to protect the circulating blood volume. Increased renal sodium reabsorption results, at least in part, from hyperaldosteronism, altered renal hemodynamics, and increased sympathetic tone. The increased water reabsorption is secondary to the nonosmotic, hypovolemic stimulus for release of antidiuretic hormone (ADH). Accordingly, the urine in prerenal disease is relatively free of sodium and water; therefore, the urine sodium concentration is less than 10 mEq/L, the fractional excretion of sodium (FE_{Na}) is less than 1%, and the urine osmolality is greater than 450 mOsm/kg water (Fig. 7-3). In addition, the ratio of BUN to serum creatinine usually exceeds 20:1 in these patients. This ratio normally is 10:1 to 15:1, but because urea reabsorption is coupled passively to sodium reabsorption in the kidney, the increase in renal sodium reabsorption in volume-depleted states, relative or absolute, is accompanied by an increase in urea reabsorption, a decline in urea clearance disproportionate to GFR alterations, and therefore, a rise in BUN. Because creatinine reabsorption is independent of sodium reabsorption, the serum creatinine does not rise by an amount out of proportion to the decline in GFR; this results in an increase in the BUN–serum creatinine ratio, which often exceeds 20:1. The selective increase in BUN in these functional renal disease states is commonly referred to as *prerenal azotemia.*

PROBLEM 1

The laboratory data from two patients with impaired renal function are provided. Which patient has acute renal failure secondary to dehydration and prerenal acute renal failure, and which patient has a chronically elevated creatinine?

  Patient 1: Plasma sodium, 140 mEq/L; plasma creatinine, 2.0 mg/dl; urine sodium, 10 mEq/L; and urine creatinine, 10 mg/dl.
  Patient 2: Plasma sodium, 140 mEq/L, plasma creatinine, 2.0 mg/dl; urine sodium, 10 mEq/L; and urine creatinine, 20 mg/dl.

ANSWER: Both patients have identical urine sodiums, and the BUN values are not provided. The FE_{Na} is therefore the only parameter that can be assessed to distinguish between these possibilities. In Chapter 2, the concept of fractional excretion was introduced. Recall that the fractional excretion can be calculated without knowing the volume of urine produced.

$$FE_{Na} = (U_{Na})(P_{Cr})/(U_{Cr})(P_{Na})$$

or

$$FE_{Na} \text{ patient } 1 = (10 \text{ mEq/L})(2 \text{ mg/dl})/(10 \text{ mg/dl})(140 \text{ mEq/L})$$
$$= .014 \text{ or } 1.4\%$$

$$FE_{Na} \text{ patient } 2 = (10 \text{ mEq/L})(2 \text{ mg/dl})/(20 \text{ mg/dl})(140 \text{ mEq/L})$$
$$= .007 \text{ or } 0.7\%$$

Patient 2 has a FE_{Na} of less than 1%, which is consistent with prerenal acute renal failure caused by dehydration. Patient 1 has a FE_{Na} of greater than 1%,

(continued)

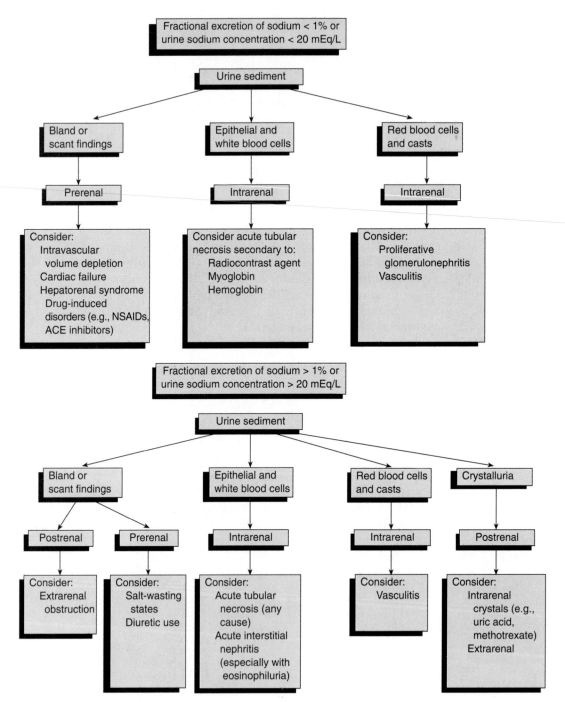

Figure 7-2. Use of urinary indices and findings in the approach to the diagnosis of acute renal failure. (ACE, angiotensin-converting enzyme; NSAIDs, nonsteroidal antiinflammatory drugs.)

which is consistent with chronic renal disease or acute renal failure secondary to intrinsic renal disease or obstruction, as discussed later in this chapter.

There are several clinical situations, however, in which these diagnostic laboratory indices may be misleading. Individuals with preexisting renal disease lose the ability to conserve sodium maximally and to concentrate the urine to levels below 10 mEq/L and above 400 mOsm/kg water, respectively. Furthermore, if volume depletion is the result of renal salt wasting, the urine sodium concentration may be high. Even in the presence of prerenal disorders, the BUN–creatinine ratio may be normal if urea production is reduced because of a low protein intake or severe liver disease. The ratio may be greater than 20:1 in obstructive renal disease, because of the enhanced urea reabsorption arising from low rates of urine flow.

Associated disturbances of plasma electrolytes also may be of diagnostic assistance in prerenal states. Volume depletion, absolute or relative, is a strong nonosmotic stimulus to ADH release, which can override the osmotic control of ADH secretion. If water ingestion exceeds water excretion in these syndromes, dilutional hyponatremia will develop. Hyponatremia and hyperuricemia may accompany plasma electrolyte abnormalities in prerenal azotemia.

Diagnostic indices in acute renal failure

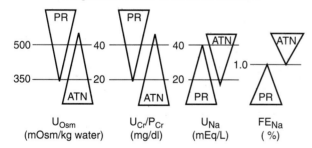

Figure 7-3. Common urinary indices in acute renal failure. The horizontal axis displays four laboratory tests and the units used to differentiate functional prerenal (PR) azotemia from acute tubular necrosis (ATN). The vertical axis depicts values that define the nondiagnostic zones of overlap between the designated values and diagnostic areas of nonoverlap above and below the designated values. The derived urinary index, the fractional excretion of sodium (FE_{Na}), has essentially no nondiagnostic overlap zone. The fraction of the filtered sodium FENa can be calculated from a urine specimen:

$$FE_{Na} \ (\%) = \frac{\text{quantity of sodium excreted}}{\text{quantity of sodium filtered}} \times 100$$

Because the quantity of sodium excreted is equal to the product of the urine sodium concentration U_{Na} and the urine volume V, the quantity of sodium filtered is equal to the product of the plasma sodium concentration (P_{Na}) and the GFR (or creatinine clearance, $C_{Cr} = U_{Cr} \times V/P_{Cr}$):

$$FE_{Na} = \frac{U_{Na} \times V}{P_{Na} \times (U_{Cr} \ V/P_{Cr})} \times 100 = \frac{U_{Na} \times P_{Cr}}{P_{Na} \times U_{Cr}} \times 100 = \left(\frac{U}{P}\right)_{Na} \times \left(\frac{P}{U}\right)_{Cr} \times 100$$

TREATMENT

The goal of therapy in prerenal acute renal failure is to improve renal perfusion. The manner in which this goal is achieved depends on the underlying disorder. The treatment of various causes of hypotension, such as hypovolemia, sepsis, and cardiac failure, is beyond the scope of this discussion. When hypovolemia from volume depletion is the cause of prerenal azotemia, infusion of saline and plasma volume expanders, preferably albumin-containing solutions, is indicated. As volume is replaced, the clinical signs of volume depletion disappear, and lowering of BUN and serum creatinine elevations develop within 12 to 24 hours; several days may be necessary to return the BUN and serum creatinine levels to baseline.

In the edematous disorders, the development of prerenal azotemia usually results from excessive diuresis and diminished intravascular volume. This diminution of intravascular volume can occur even though peripheral edema and elevated total body sodium content persist in the patient. In these circumstances, gentle volume repletion will improve renal functional parameters. Care must be used not to overzealously expand intravascular volume and run the risk of greater edema formation and congestive heart failure. Treatment should also be directed toward the underlying disease process. Cardiac failure can be treated with digitalis and vasodilators: Some forms of nephrotic syndrome are responsive to corticosteroids (see Chap. 5). The presence of prerenal azotemia in a patient with congestive heart failure that is not the result of overdiuresis is usually reflective of severe cardiac dysfunction and demands special attention to improve cardiac reserve.

ACUTE RENAL FAILURE SECONDARY TO INTRINSIC RENAL PROCESSES

Intrarenal processes are the most common causes of acute renal failure. *Acute tubular necrosis* (ATN), arising from either ischemic or toxic events, dominates this category, although immunologic processes, including glomerulonephritis, interstitial nephritis, and vascular diseases, also must be considered in the differential diagnosis.

ACUTE TUBULAR NECROSIS

Although ATN represents a nonspecific response to a variety of insults, including ischemia and endogenous and exogenous toxins, there are similarities in the pathology, pathophysiology, clinical course, diagnosis, and treatment of this renal disorder, regardless of the etiology.

Pathophysiology

Acute tubular necrosis occurs from tubular injury that produces only segmental necrosis in tubular elements within the kidney. In most cases, a very patchy distribution of frankly necrotic lesions appears to be the rule rather than the exception, as seen in Figure 7-4. Because loss of renal tubular cell integrity and function is the primary pathogenetic event in either ischemic or nephrotoxic acute renal failure, ATN continues to be the most acceptable term to describe this complex clinical disorder. In this chapter, the terms ATN and acute renal failure derived from ischemic or nephrotoxic insults are used interchangeably.

The final common pathogenic pathway for the development of acute renal

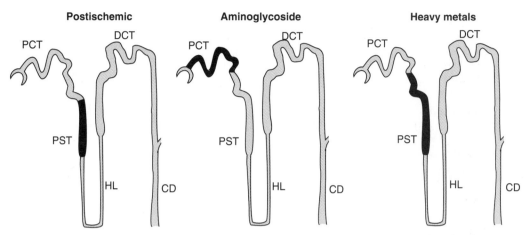

Figure 7-4. The patchy, segmental distribution of tubular cell necrosis in postischemic and nephrotoxic acute renal failure. The proximal straight tubule (PST) segments are most vulnerable to ischemia and heavy metal toxicity. The proximal convoluted tubule segments (PCT) are most susceptible to aminoglycoside toxicity. In both nephrotoxic and ischemic injury, the lumina of distal segments of the nephrons are occupied by casts. (CD, collecting duct; DCT, distal convoluted tubule; HL, Henle's loop.

failure, be it ischemic or nephrotoxic in origin, is renal tubular cell injury. Progressive renal tubular cell injury initiates alterations at the nephronal level that ultimately result in renal excretory failure, as shown in Figure 7-5. These alterations are tubular obstruction and backleak of glomerular filtrate through damaged tubular epithelium. Intratubular obstruction appears to be a major nephronal mechanism for a GFR decline in ATN. Clinicians are well aware of the potential for obstruction to the flow of urine at the level of the ureters, or beyond, along the

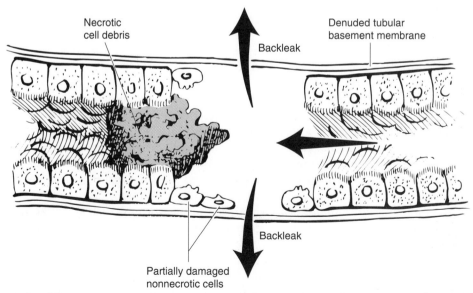

Figure 7-5. The pathophysiology of acute tubular necrosis (ATN). Intratubular obstruction from cell debris and backleak of glomerular filtrate across the denuded basement membrane are the major nephronal mechanisms for a GFR decline in ATN.

urinary collecting system, to result in acute renal failure. Intratubular blockage of urine flow can result in similar decreases in renal excretory function if the blockage is diffuse enough to involve most functioning nephrons. Casts made up of cellular debris from injured or necrotic renal tubule cells are frequently found in the distal nephron, where they impede the flow of urine. The necrotic cells shed into the tubular lumen reduce renal excretory function not only by obstructing urine flow but also by leaving gaps along the tubular epithelia through which glomerular filtrate can reenter the circulation, a process termed *backleak of glomerular filtrate.*

Etiology

The etiology of ATN can be divided into two major categories: postischemic and nephrotoxic. In many clinical settings, a combination of these two processes operate simultaneously to produce acute renal failure. An ischemic insult often potentiates renal damage produced by nephrotoxins.

Renal ischemia is the most common cause of ATN. There is a large variability in the length and severity of the ischemic insults that produce ischemic acute renal failure in clinical settings. In some patients, a few minutes of ischemia produces ATN, whereas in others, prolonged renal ischemia produces only transient renal dysfunction. The reason for this variation is not known. Any prerenal cause of renal excretory function, if prolonged and severe enough, can eventuate in the progression to structural renal damage. Most cases of ischemic acute renal failure, however, are associated with a period of frank hypotension. Postischemic acute renal failure is seen with higher frequency in patients with sepsis or those undergoing major surgery.

Nearly one half of the clinical cases of ischemic acute renal failure follow surgery. A variety of processes, including preoperative and intraoperative fluid losses and anesthesia, result in intravascular volume depletion, causing declines in RBF and GFR. If an additional hypotensive or hemolytic insult is added to these conditions, susceptible patients may develop ATN. Abdominal aortic aneurysmal repair, open heart surgery, and biliary tract surgery are the surgical procedures with the highest incidence of postischemic acute renal failure. Each of these procedures is associated with a substantially greater decline in RBF than other surgical procedures. This tendency may relate to stimulation of neural inputs to the kidney, which control renal arteriolar tone and are activated by manipulation of the biliary tract, abdominal aorta, and heart. The higher frequency of ATN in the septic patient may relate to the major hemodynamic effects of endotoxins that have the ability to produce hypotension and substantial renal vasoconstriction.

Because the kidney is a major excretory organ of the body for therapeutic agents, the list of drugs that can induce *nephrotoxic acute renal failure* is long. As new agents are developed, additions to this list certainly will be made. The causes for nephrotoxic acute renal failure can be categorized into four major groups: antibiotics, heavy metals, radiocontrast agents, and endogenous toxins (Table 7-2).

Aminoglycoside antibiotics are a mainstay of therapy in the clinical treatment of gram-negative infections. Because gram-negative organisms account for the majority of hospital-acquired infections, the occurrence of aminoglycoside-induced acute renal failure has become commonplace. Approximately 10% of patients receiving parenteral therapy with aminoglycosides develop significant declines in GFR. Several aminoglycoside antibiotics are available clinically, including neomycin, gentamicin, tobramycin, kanamycin, amikacin, netilmicin, and streptomycin.

TABLE 7-2. *CAUSES OF ACUTE TUBULAR NECROSIS*

Postischemic acute tubular necrosis

Nephrotoxic acute tubular necrosis

    Antibiotics (e.g., aminoglycosides, amphotericin B)

    Heavy metals (e.g., cis-platin)

    Radiocontrast agents

    Cyclosporine

    Endogenous toxins (e.g., myoglobin, hemoglobin, light chains)

The kidney is the principal excretory route for the elimination of the aminoglycoside antibiotics, which results in the accumulation of these antibiotics in the renal cortex. Aminoglycosides produce tubular cell necrosis that is confined exclusively to the proximal tubule. Aminoglycoside nephrotoxicity is associated classically with a nonoliguric type of acute renal failure; excretory failure may develop in the presence of normal urinary outputs of 1 to 2 L/day. Urinary output is, therefore, an unreliable marker for detecting aminoglycoside nephrotoxicity. Declines in effective GFR and elevations in serum creatinine usually are not seen clinically prior to 5 to 7 days of aminoglycoside treatment.

A variety of factors are known to predispose to aminoglycoside nephrotoxicity, most importantly, the *dose and duration of drug administration.* Higher antibiotic doses result in higher serum drug levels and more rapid aminoglycoside accumulation in the kidney. *Prolonged therapy* increases the risk of achieving toxic concentrations within renal parenchyma. The risk of developing this clinical disorder is increased not only in patients given continuous and prolonged therapy but also in those given repeated courses of an aminoglycoside separated by a few days or weeks. Preexisting renal insufficiency is another important risk factor and has been shown to increase the rate of aminoglycoside nephrotoxicity, perhaps because toxin load per residual functioning nephron is greater in patients with renal insufficiency compared with those in the normal state.

In addition to aminoglycosides, other antibiotics have been associated with nephrotoxicity, including amphotericin B. This agent is the most effective antibiotic agent for the treatment of deep-seated and disseminated fungal infections. Amphotericin B is a polyene antibiotic that exerts its effects on microorganisms by interacting with the lipid sterols present in the outer membranes of susceptible cells. Bacteria, which lack sterols as components of their membranes, are not affected by polyenes. Fungi, however, contain ergosterol as part of their membranes, and they lose their surface integrity after exposure to polyene antibiotics. Similarly, mammalian cells that possess cholesterol are also disrupted by polyenes. Renal toxicity is a major side effect of this agent. The decline in GFR is related acutely to this drug's effect to promote renal vascular vasoconstriction and a diminution of renal blood flow, with chronic administration renal tubular cell damage.

A variety of *heavy metals* produce acute renal failure with proximal tubular necrosis. Salts of mercury, platinum, arsenic, bismuth, silver, chromium, and uranium are very potent nephrotoxins. ATN secondary to these agents is almost completely confined to occupational exposure or ingestion, either accidental or purposeful. Of the heavy metals, platinum in the form of the inorganic compound cis-diamminedichloroplatinum, or simply *cis-platin,* is the predominant causes of heavy metal nephrotoxicity in clinical settings. Cis-platin is one of a class of platinum derivatives that has proved effective against certain solid tumors. As with other nephrotoxic agents, the incidence of renal toxicity associated with cis-platin is dependent on dose.

A significant increase in the incidence of *radiocontrast-induced ATN* has occurred recently. This increased over the past several years is attributable to the greater use of these agents for an increasing number of radiologic procedures, including intravenous pyelography (IVP), angiography, and computered tomography (CT).

Because the kidney is the principal excretory organ for these compounds, the potential exists for nephrotoxicity to occur with their use. The incidence of nephrotoxicity is relatively low for urographic and CT scanning procedures. Because of the larger doses required, angiography may have a slightly higher incidence of toxic reactions in the kidney. Certain clinical risk factors may increase this incidence, especially preexisting renal insufficiency and long-standing insulin-dependent diabetes mellitus. Other less critical risk factors include volume depletion, contrast dose, and multiple myeloma. This form of nephrotoxic ATN can present with an FE_{Na} of less than 1%.

CASE 2

A 63-year-old male executive is admitted for an elective cardiac catheterization to evaluate exertional chest pain. The patient has had essential hypertension for 12 years; blood pressure is controlled with thiazides and β-blockers. He has a history of insulin-dependent diabetes for 14 years but no evidence of diabetic neuropathy, retinopathy, nephropathy, or enteropathy. A recent 24-hour urinary protein excretion was quantitated at 1.7 g. His admission laboratory values reveal normal electrolytes, a BUN of 26 mg/dl, and a serum creatinine level of 1.6 mg/dl. Urinalysis is unremarkable. Previous workup suggests that the modest decline in renal function is most consistent with nephrosclerosis. The next day he undergoes cardiac catheterization, which is complicated by difficulty in placing the catheter into one of the coronary arteries and required multiple attempts and multiple injections of contrast material. Following the procedure, the nursing staff realizes the patient has had no urine output during the next 18 hours. Catheterization of the urinary bladder produced 100 ml of urine that had a U_{Na} of 5 mEq/L, a FE_{Na} of 0.9% and multiple granular casts and renal tubular epithelial cells in the spun sediment. The patient has an abdominal x-ray film demonstrating a persistent nephrogram. His oliguria persists over the next 3 days, with his BUN and serum creatinine rising to levels of 45 and 4.2 mg/dl, respectively. Over the ensuing 10 days, his urine output gradually increases and his renal function parameters return to baseline values.

CASE DISCUSSION

The patient has two significant risk factors for the development of radiocontrast-induced acute renal failure: insulin-dependent diabetes mellitus and renal insufficiency. The study was definitely indicated, but the contrast load was high because of technical difficulties with the catheterization. To lessen the risk of toxicity, the patient should have been well hydrated with saline solution overnight prior to the procedure. The diagnosis is relatively easy because of timing between contrast administration and oliguria, low FE_{Na}, abnormal urine sediment, and persistent nephrogram. Fortunately, the degree of renal insult is mild to moderate and reversibility occurs prior to uremic symptomatology. Consequently, dialysis is not needed.

Endogenous toxins, including myoglobin, hemoglobin, and myeloma light chains, can cause acute renal failure. Large amounts of *myoglobin* are contained in muscle tissue. Muscle damage results in the release of myoglobin, which, because it is a low-molecular-weight protein, is filterable and excreted in the urine. Myoglobinuric acute renal failure most often develops from traumatic muscle injury. Some forms of multiple myeloma, a form of plasma cell leukemia, are associated with high production of circulating *immunoglobulin light chains*, which have potential properties to induce nephrotoxic damage to renal tubule cells or interact with urinary proteins to produce intratubular obstructing casts. Accordingly, acute renal failure can be an accompanying disorder with this form of malignancy.

CASE 3

A 24-year-old known intravenous drug abuser is found unconscious in his room and is brought to the emergency department. It is unknown how long he has been unconscious or what drugs he has been taking. He does not respond to the administration of narcotic antagonists. On physical examination, he is obtunded, but his vital signs are normal. No evidence of trauma is present. A urinary bladder catheter is placed, and 150 ml of dark urine is collected. The urine and the supernatant of the spun urine are both positive for heme by dipstick. The urine sediment reveals pigmented granular casts and numerous renal tubular epithelial cells but no red blood cells or white blood cells. The plasma obtained from the patient is not pink. Laboratory values reveal the following values: normal serum sodium, 137 mEq/L; potassium, 5.9 mEq/L; chloride, 99 mEq/L; bicarbonate, 21 mEq/L; serum calcium, 6.0 mg/dl; serum albumin, 4.1 g/dl; serum phosphate, 9.8 mg/dl; uric acid, 16.3 mg/dl; serum creatinine, 2.6 mg/dl; BUN, 19 mg/dl; and serum creatinine phosphokinase, 12,800 U/ml. The urine is sent for toxicologic screen and myoglobin determination.

CASE DISCUSSION

This patient presents with oliguria. The dark urine, which is heme-positive on dipstick, together with the absence of red blood cells in the urine sediment, suggests heme pigment–induced acute renal failure. Because myoglobin is a smaller molecule than hemoglobin, the plasma is usually clear with myoglobinuria because of rapid renal clearance but pink with hemoglobinuria. The hyperkalemia, hypocalcemia, hyperphosphatemia, hyperuricemia, low BUN–serum creatinine ratio (7:1 in this case), and elevated creatinine phosphokinase values all suggest rhabdomyolytic myoglobinuric ATN. This disorder is occasionally seen in intravenous drug abusers and is the result of myonecrosis from pressure and ischemic stress, as is the case in this patient.

Diagnosis

Before a diagnosis of ATN can be made, prerenal and postrenal causes of renal insufficiency must be excluded.

History. After other causes of acute renal failure have been excluded, a detailed investigation must be undertaken to identify causes of ischemic and nephrotoxic ATN. Careful review of the patient's clinical course before the development of acute renal failure is necessary. Special attention should be given to the temporal relation of fluid and electrolyte abnormalities, volume status, blood pressure, medication administration, surgical procedures, potential nephrotoxin exposure, and renal function parameters just before the development of ATN. This is particularly true for aminoglycoside, amphotericin B, cisplatin, and radiocontrast-associated nephrotoxicity.

Laboratory Tests. Key urinary findings may aid in the correct diagnosis (see Figs. 7-2 and 7-3). The urine sediment in the early phase of ATN usually contains renal tubular epithelial cells and granular and epithelial cell casts. Because tubular function is impaired, the kidney's ability to conserve sodium and maximally concentrate the urine is diminished. These abnormalities can be of diagnostic value in patients with azotemia in differentiating between prerenal azotemia and ATN (see Fig. 7-3). In patients whose azotemia is secondary to prerenal causes, the urinary indices usually show a urinary osmolality greater than 500 mOsm/kg water, a urinary sodium concentration less than 10 mEq/L, and a urine–plasma creatinine ratio less than 20. Although these ranges in urinary indices are diagnostic in approximately 80% of patients, approximately 20% have indices in an intermediate, nondiagnostic zone. Further discrimination between these two causes of azotemia can be made by use of the derived fractional sodium excretion (FE_{Na}) index, which is greater than 1% in patients with ATN and less than 1% in patients with prerenal azotemia. Patients with radiocontrast-induced acute renal failure often have FE_{Na} values less than 1% even though ATN is present. The reason for this phenomenon is not known. Because nephrotoxic ATN is becoming the most common cause of acute renal failure in the clinical setting, knowledge of the large number of drugs possessing nephrotoxic potential will be of substantial benefit in establishing the correct diagnosis.

Treatment

The therapy of ATN is to prevent or ameliorate renal injury during the developing phase of acute renal failure and to treat established disease during the renal failure and recovery phases of ATN. Prevention of ischemic acute renal failure is primarily directed toward maintaining adequate renal perfusion. Because volume depletion increases the risk of ischemic ATN following surgery and sepsis, careful attention should be directed toward maintenance of euvolemia in patients at risk.

Nephrotoxic acute renal failure is also best handled by prevention. Prevention, however, requires a knowledge of the drugs that possess nephrotoxic side effects and their correct dosage, the careful and deliberate selection of these nephrotoxic agents only for clearly defined clinical indications, and the identification and modulation of the factors that increase the risk of nephrotoxic complications. The preceding section includes comments on each of these areas for each group of drugs but, as a general approach to prevention, several specific risk factors that predispose a patient to develop renal complications from most drugs with nephrotoxic potential can be identified.

Nephrotoxic agents are nephrotoxic because they are excreted from the body primarily by the kidneys. *Preexisting renal dysfunction*, therefore, results in longer serum half-lives of the drugs and a greater time to interact deleteriously with renal cells and their membrane components. Dosage adjustments are imperative in these patients. Furthermore, with renal dysfunction, the number of functioning nephrons declines, and the load of excreted drug per nephron rises proportionately. Therefore, a toxic level at the nephronal level can be achieved more easily in patients with preexisting renal disease. Thus, the renal cell in a kidney with diminished function has the potential, if dosage adjustments are not made, to be exposed to higher, potentially toxic, drug concentrations for longer time periods than the renal cell in a kidney with normal function.

Volume depletion results in avid sodium and water reabsorption along the proximal tubule and the collecting duct of the nephron. Because the handling of most compounds, including drugs, by the kidney is profoundly affected by alterations in sodium transport, the nephronal alterations in the handling of sodium and water in a volume-depleted state may result either in greater intratubular concentrations, which may be frankly toxic to plasma membranes, or in increased renal tubular cell transport of the drug into its intracellular environment and greater intracellular levels which may approach toxic concentrations. Volume repletion and euvolemia are important conditions to maintain during nephrotoxic drug administration.

Because endogenous creatinine production is dependent on muscle mass, and muscle mass declines with age, a normal or slightly elevated level of serum creatinine in an *elderly individual* may reflect a much lower creatinine clearance, or GFR, than that of a young individual with an identical level of serum creatinine. Therefore, elderly patients may have more profound preexisting renal disease than can be appreciated by the level of serum creatinine.

Even with the careful use of nephrotoxic agents, renal toxicity will occur occasionally. When objective evidence of declines in GFR develops with a rising level of serum creatinine and BUN, the drug or drugs that may be responsible for nephrotoxicity should be discontinued if possible. Even after the drug responsible for renal damage is withdrawn, renal dysfunction may progress for several days, because toxic injury continues from the persistence of the toxin within the renal parenchyma. Careful monitoring of renal function is therefore necessary even after recognition of the insult.

Once ischemic or nephrotoxic acute renal failure occurs, its treatment is similar to that of acute renal failure from other processes. The basic goals are the maintenance of fluid and electrolyte balance, adequate nutrition, and when present, treatment of infection and uremia. The use of mannitol or furosemide is controversial in the treatment of ATN. There is no good evidence that the use of these diuretic agents can reverse ATN once it has developed. The use of these agents can convert an occasional patient from oliguric to nonoliguric ATN. Because nonoliguric ATN is more manageable clinically and may have a lower mortality rate, these agents may be considered for this indication. If there is no response of increased urine flow, however, multiple doses should be avoided, because the retention of hypertonic mannitol in the extracellular space can result in hyperosmolality, hyponatremia, extracellular fluid overload, and possibly pulmonary edema. Deafness, which can be irreversible, can follow the use of large doses of furosemide or, more commonly, ethacrynic acid.

Some patients, usually those with oliguric ATN, require dialysis. Either peritoneal dialysis or hemodialysis can be used. Strict indications for dialysis are an inability to control hyperkalemia with cation-exchange resins, particularly in hypercatabolic states, which release large amounts of intracellular potassium to the extracellular space; fluid overload; and the uremic complications of pericarditis and encephalopathy. If the patient is oliguric with steadily rising levels of serum creatinine, dialysis usually is initiated when the level of serum creatinine reaches 8 to 10 mg/100 ml to avoid major uremic problems, which rapidly would become life-threatening. Furthermore, maintenance of levels of BUN below 100 mg/100 ml may improve the general condition of the patient by limiting uremia-related impairment of white blood cell and platelet function.

The prognosis of patients with ATN depends on the etiology of the condition. ATN following surgery or trauma has an overall mortality rate of 40% to 75%. The survival rate is much better among those patients who do not develop other medical complications, such as infection, bleeding, or respiratory failure. Patients with nephrotoxic ATN have an average mortality rate of less than 10%. Because dialysis is able to correct most abnormalities associated with renal excretory failure, the dependence of patient survival on extrarenal disturbances is not surprising.

Clinical Course

The decline in renal function observed in ATN can begin abruptly after an ischemic event or develop insidiously from nephrotoxic injury. The daily increases in BUN and serum creatinine vary between 10 and 25 mg/dl and 0.5 and 2.5 mg/dl, respectively. The clinical problems that can occur during the developing phase of renal failure include: volume overload; electrolyte disorders, such as hyponatremia, hyperkalemia, hyperphosphatemia, hypocalcemia, and acidemia; and signs and symptoms of uremia, including pericarditis, lethargy, vomiting, and infection. The renal failure predisposes the patient to develop infectious complications because of poor white cell chemotaxis, reduced reticuloendothelial clearance, and diminished lymphocytic responsiveness to antigens. Infection is the most common cause of death in uremia.

During this phase, the patient usually is oliguric; however, urine outputs greater than 500 ml/day, or nonoliguria, may develop in 30% to 40% of patients with ATN. The urine output therefore cannot and should not be used as an accurate reflection of GFR in developing ATN. It appears that nonoliguric ATN has a better prognosis than oliguric ATN. This better natural history is, at least in part, the consequence of a lesser incidence of hyperkalemia and fluid overload. A more probable reason for this clinical observation is the fact that nonoliguric renal failure is a reflection of lesser degrees of renal damage, with less frequent progression to symptomatic renal failure requiring dialysis.

Renal excretory failure persists for an average of 7 to 21 days. At times, ATN may result in irreversible renal failure, particularly in the clinical setting, where it is of multifactorial origin in the critically ill patient. The potential reversibility is the result of the regenerative ability of surviving renal epithelial cells. Necrotic areas are replaced with new functional cells. Renal function can return completely, or nearly completely, to baseline levels. As renal function improves, urine output increases, and serum creatinine levels decline. During the course of acute renal failure, serum creatinine concentration typically follows a *triphasic pattern*, as demonstrated in Figure 7-6. In the developing phase of ATN, serum creatinine concentration progressively increases. During the early recovery phase, the im-

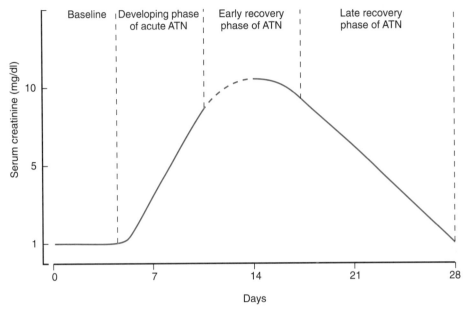

Figure 7-6. Typical triphasic change in serum creatinine concentration during developing, early recovery, and late recovery phases of acute tubular necrosis (ATN). During the early recovery period, the serum creatinine concentration may still rise as the glomerular filtration rate improves. The rate of change in serum creatinine, however, will be less (*dashed lines*).

provements in GFR increase creatinine excretion. As the rate of creatinine excretion approaches the rate of creatinine production, the daily increases in serum creatinine become smaller. Thus, even with an improvement in GFR, serum creatinine still may increase for several days. With further improvement in GFR, creatinine excretion exceeds production, so that serum creatinine finally reaches a plateau and gradually declines back toward normal.

ACUTE RENAL FAILURE SECONDARY TO OBSTRUCTIVE CAUSES

Obstruction of urine flow may occur at any site along the urinary tract. Acute renal failure from obstructive disease occurs from extrarenal processes (Table 7-3). In the approach to renal diseases in general, because extrarenal urinary tract obstruction is a reversible cause of renal failure, urinary tract obstruction always should be considered as part of the initial differential diagnosis in every patient who presents with renal insufficiency.

INTRARENAL OBSTRUCTION

Acute renal failure can arise secondary to intrarenal obstruction from crystal formation and precipitation occurring diffusely within tubular lumina throughout the kidney. Because most cases of intrarenal obstructive acute renal failure present similarly to those from other causes of ATN and result from intrarenal rather than extrarenal obstruction, the diagnosis is not made with the commonly used urologic procedures of cystoscopy or retrograde pyelography. Usually, the diagnosis is made

TABLE 7-3. *EXTRARENAL CAUSES OF OBSTRUCTIVE ACUTE RENAL FAILURE*

Intrarenal
    Acute uric acid nephropathy
Extrarenal
    Renal pelvis: calculus, sloughed papilla, ureteropelvic junction
    Ureter: lymphoma, neoplasia (ureteral, prostate, bladder, pelvis), calculus, sloughed papilla, pregnancy, stricture
    Urethra and bladder neck: benign prostatic hypertrophy, neoplasia (prostate, bladder), neurogenic bladder, calculus

because of an awareness of the settings in which intrarenal crystal formation and precipitation can develop.

Acute uric acid nephropathy is commonly seen with the use of a variety of chemotherapeutic agents in patients with myeloproliferative or lymphoproliferative disorders. Treatment results in the rapid destruction of neoplastic tissue and the elaboration of uric acid from the nucleic acids released from lysed cells, followed by hyperuricemia, uricosuria, precipitation of uric acid crystals intrarenally, and acute renal failure. Clinically, this disorder is characterized by the acute onset of oliguria, often leading to anuria with rapidly rising levels of BUN and creatinine. The level of serum uric acid usually exceeds 20 mg/100 ml. In the early phase, uric acid crystals and hematuria are commonly found in the urinalysis. A uric acid–creatinine concentration ratio greater than 1 on a random urine sample may aid in the diagnosis.

Treatment is directed toward minimizing the occurrence of uric acid crystal formation within the collecting ducts of the kidney. Since the pK_a of uric acid is 5.75, raising urine pH and increasing the urine flow rate favor excretion of urate salts. Urinary alkalinization is induced by infusion of sodium bicarbonate and concomitant administration of the carbonic anhydrase inhibitor acetazolamide. In patients with acute leukemia for whom combination chemotherapy is planned, pretreatment with allopurinol for at least 24 hours, and preferably for 3 days diminishes the hyperuricemic response and the risk of this disorder. In patients with established renal failure or serum uric acid levels exceeding 25 mg/100 ml, hemodialysis is indicated to lower serum uric acid and to reverse the acute renal failure. Rare cases of this form of acute renal failure have been reported with other drugs, including the diuretic ticrynafen, the chemotherapeutic agent methotrexate, and the sulfanamide antibiotics.

EXTRARENAL OBSTRUCTION

Extrarenal obstruction to urine flow can occur at the level of the renal pelvis, ureter, urethra, or bladder neck. A wide variety of processes may cause urinary tract obstruction. In young adults, renal stones are the major cause of obstruction. In older adults, prostatic hypertrophy, various neoplasms, and renal stones are the most common causes of extrarenal obstruction.

CASE 4

A 72-year-old man with long-standing dementia is transferred from a local nursing home because of fever. On physical examination, he has stable vital signs but a temperature of 39°C. He does not appear volume-depleted. His lungs are clear and his abdominal examination benign. His admitting laboratory values are as follows: serum Na⁺, 138 mEq/L; Cl⁻, 100 mEq/L; K⁺, 6.2 mEq/L; HCO₃⁻, 19 mEq/L; BUN, 100 mg/dl; and serum creatinine, 6.2 mg/dl. The patient has no urine output over the next 4 hours. A urinary bladder catheter is passed with difficulty and drains 600 ml of urine, at which time it is clamped. Over the next 3 hours, a total of 2000 ml of urine is collected with intermittent clamping. The urinalysis demonstrates 10 to 20 white blood cells/high power field and gram-negative organisms on Gram stain. He is begun on antibiotics and shows clinical improvement. Over the subsequent 8 hours, the patient has 2000 ml of urine output, which is replaced with 1000 ml of saline solution. His urine output gradually tapers, and his BUN and creatinine fall to 25 and 1.4 mg/dl, respectively, over the next 3 days.

CASE DISCUSSION

This patient presented with unknown etiology of renal failure, so that prerenal, intrarenal, and postrenal causes had to be entertained in the differential diagnosis. Fortunately, urinary bladder neck obstruction, most likely secondary to prostatic hypertrophy, is diagnosed and treated with placement of a bladder catheter. Complete drainage is not accomplished immediately but is achieved over several hours to prevent a possible hypotensive response. The urinary tract obstruction is accompanied by a urinary tract infection, which requires both antibiotics and drainage for treatment. The patient has a moderate postobstructive diuresis, which is conservatively replaced with parenteral fluids. Over the ensuing hospital course, his renal function returns to near-normal levels.

When the obstructive process is acute, suprapubic or flank pain is common. The location of the pain is determined by the site of obstruction. If the process is slowly progressive and chronic or intrarenal, there may be no symptoms. The urinalysis may be entirely normal, but crystals and hematuria may be present if the renal failure is caused by intratubular crystal deposition or passage of stones. A normal or even high urine output can be seen in obstructive uropathy. Although complete obstruction results in anuria, intermittent and partial urinary tract obstruction can result in marked declines in GFR in the presence of intermittent and variable urine outputs.

In addition to the signs and symptoms directly referable to obstruction, it is important to look for underlying disorders that may be the cause of the obstruction. Clues to the cause may be provided by a history of malignancy; previous abdominal, pelvic, or genitourinary surgery; renal stones; disorders associated with papillary necrosis (e.g., diabetes mellitus, analgesic nephropathy, sickle cell disease); or treatment with methysergide, a drug that is used for the treatment of migraine headache and can cause retroperitoneal fibrosis.

A variety of complications can develop with urinary tract obstruction. With urinary stasis, infection develops more frequently. Hypertension occasionally develops in patients with urinary tract obstruction and appears to be volume-related. Renal failure develops only with bilateral obstruction, or with unilateral obstruction in the case of a solitary kidney. Papillary necrosis also may develop with acute obstruction and appears to have an ischemic basis.

The diagnosis of urinary tract obstruction begins with a high degree of suspicion, and the evaluation of a suspected obstruction begins with catheterization of the urinary bladder. If urethral obstruction or neurogenic bladder is the cause, urine output will increase. Because the rapid removal of a large urinary volume in the relief of obstruction has been at times associated with hypotension, only 500 ml should be initially removed. The remainder of urine can than be drained over several hours, with intermittent clamping of the drainage catheter.

If bladder catheterization does not result in a vigorous urine output, the obstruction must be at the level of the ureters or higher. In these cases, the diagnosis of obstruction depends on radiologic procedures, including ultrasonography, IVP, CT scanning, or retrograde pyelography. Because of the decline in renal function, IVP visualization of the collecting system in obstruction might not occur until 6 to 24 hours after dye administration.

The necessity and rapidity of treatment of urinary tract obstruction depends on the clinical setting and on whether the obstruction is complete or partial. Immediate relief of obstruction is necessary only in patients with generalized sepsis as a result of infection proximal to the obstruction. Antibiotic therapy alone in this setting is usually ineffective. Pain, recurrent infections or bleeding, or progressive impairment in renal function are other indications for correction of obstruction, but immediate therapy is not required. A short delay in relieving the obstruction will not lead to irreversible deterioration in renal function. Complete restoration of renal function can occur if the obstruction is corrected within 1 week of onset. If obstruction persists for 1 to 4 weeks, some permanent loss of function occurs, although the GFR may return to 30% to 50% of normal. After 5 to 12 weeks of complete obstruction, only 10% of renal function can return.

The particular therapeutic intervention for relief of urinary tract obstruction depends on the site and cause of the obstruction. The relief of bilateral complete urinary tract obstruction is often associated with a period of high urine output, referred to as *postobstructive diuresis*. In most patients, this diuresis is appropriate and represents the loss of fluid retained during the period of complete obstruction. Rarely, the diuresis is inappropriate, resulting in volume depletion if the urine output is not replaced. The recommended approach to postobstructive diuresis is to allow the patient to develop negative fluid balance by not replacing all fluid losses unless signs of volume depletion occur. In this manner, the ongoing diuresis is not maintained iatrogenically.

SELECTED READING

Brenner BM, Lazarus JM, eds. Acute renal failure. 2nd ed. New York: Churchill Livingstone, 1988.

Humes HD. Aminoglycoside nephrotoxicity. Kidney Int 1988;33:900.

Myers BD, Moran SM. Acute renal failure. N Engl J Med 1986;314:96.

Lippincott's Pathophysiology Series: Renal Pathophysiology, edited by James A. Shayman. J. B. Lippincott Company, Philadelphia © 1995.

Chronic Renal Failure

Eric W. Young

OBJECTIVES

By the end of this chapter the reader should be able to:

- Understand the definition and implications of chronic renal failure, azotemia, uremia, and end-stage renal disease.
- List the major etiologic causes of chronic renal failure
- Understand the short-term adaptive responses that maintain kidney function after renal injury.
- Understand how these short-term adaptations can accelerate the progression of chronic renal failure.
- Understand the rationale for slowing the progression of chronic renal failure using blood pressure reduction, angiotensin-converting enzyme inhibitors, and dietary protein restriction.
- Recognize the metabolic consequences of chronic renal failure as regards sodium and water handling, potassium handling, acid–base status, mineral metabolism, drug handling, and renal endocrine function.
- Recognize the clinical consequences of chronic renal failure for the various organ systems.
- Understand the basic management principles for chronic renal failure and end-stage renal disease.

Chronic renal failure (CRF) is a clinical syndrome arising from irreversible, usually progressive, kidney injury. Many distinct pathologic entities can lead to chronic renal failure. Although the causes of CRF are diverse, the clinical course is predictable. This chapter discusses the major causes, common pathophysiologic patterns, clinical manifestations, and treatment of CRF.

CRF implies permanent injury to the kidney; the normal renal architecture is gradually replaced by scar tissue. CRF is irreversible and often progressive. In contrast, acute renal failure is often reversible, and the underlying renal architecture is usually preserved. The hallmark of renal failure is elevation of the creatinine and blood urea nitrogen (BUN) concentrations in the extracellular fluid caused by a fall in the glomerular filtration rate (GFR). Other functions of the kidney also usually are impaired, such as synthesis of renal hormones. A wide range of symptoms, signs, and laboratory alterations accompany various degrees of renal failure.

Several terms are used to describe chronic renal injury. CRF is the general term used to describe irreversible loss of GFR over a prolonged period of time, usually years. *Chronic renal insufficiency* implies mild CRF, although the degree of renal failure for this designation is not well defined. *Azotemia* refers to an elevation in the BUN and creatinine levels and does not imply any symptoms or overt clinical manifestations of kidney disease. Azotemia occurs with both chronic and acute renal failure. *Uremia* is the symptomatic phase of renal failure during which symptoms and signs of renal dysfunction are detected. For many individuals, uremic manifestations do not appear until the GFR is less than 10 ml/minute (normal, 120 ml/minute). *End-stage renal disease* (ESRD) refers to any form of chronic (i.e., irreversible) renal failure at a stage that permanent renal replacement therapy is indicated in the form of dialysis or kidney transplantation.

CAUSES OF CHRONIC RENAL FAILURE

Many different types of kidney diseases can result in CRF, just as many different types of heart disease (e.g., ischemic, valvular, myopathic) can cause congestive heart failure. An approximation of the causes of CRF can be made from the frequency of primary renal diagnoses in patients starting dialysis (Table 8-1). More

TABLE 8-1. *ATTRIBUTED CAUSES OF END-STAGE RENAL DISEASE IN THE UNITED STATES*

CAUSES OF RENAL DISEASE	PERCENT OF CASES
Diabetes	34.2
Hypertension (nephrosclerosis)	29.4
Glomerulonephritis	14.2
Interstitial nephritis	3.4
Cystic kidney disease	3.4
Other or unknown	15.4

From US Renal Data Systems, USRDS Annual Report, The National Institutes of Health, National Institute of Diabetes, Digestive, and Kidney Diseases, Bethesda, Maryland, 1993.

detailed information about most of these specific causes can be found in other sections of this book.

Diabetes is currently the most common cause of CRF leading to ESRD. Approximately one third of patients with insulin-dependent diabetes (i.e., ketosis-prone or type I diabetes) will develop diabetic nephropathy, the general term for renal disease associated with diabetes. Many patients with non–insulin-dependent diabetes also develop kidney disease. Pathologically, the kidneys show nodular or diffuse sclerosis of the glomeruli. Renal disease generally develops in patients who have had diabetes for at least 10 years, and most patients also have diabetic complications involving the eyes (i.e., diabetic retinopathy) and peripheral sensory nerves (i.e., diabetic neuropathy). The first evidence of renal disease is the appearance of small amounts of albumin in the urine, referred to as microalbuminuria because of the small quantity rather than the size of the molecule. Eventually, albuminuria progresses and can reach the nephrotic range (i.e., >3.5 g/day of protein). Azotemia develops soon after proteinuria begins and progresses to uremia and ESRD within 2 to 7 years.

Hypertension is the attributed cause of ESRD in approximately 30% of patients. Hypertension causes renal injury that is manifest as thickening of renal arterioles, a process known as nephrosclerosis. The clinical syndrome consists of slowly progressive renal failure, low-grade proteinuria, and a bland urine sediment. Kidney disease can also cause new hypertension or exacerbate preexisting hypertension. In a patient with CRF and hypertension, it is often unclear which entity caused the other. Although definitive evidence is lacking, it appears that antihypertensive treatment decreases renal damage.

Glomerulonephritis is the third most common attributed cause of ESRD. A large variety of primary and secondary glomerulonephritides can culminate in ESRD, including membranous nephropathy, focal glomerular sclerosis, systemic lupus erythematosus, and Goodpasture's syndrome (see Chaps. 5 and 6).

The remaining causes of ESRD consist of several relatively less common renal diseases. *Polycystic kidney disease* is a genetic disorder with autosomal dominant inheritance. Although polycystic kidney disease accounts for only 3.4% of ESRD cases, it is the most common genetic disease recognized. *Chronic interstitial nephritis* can occur as a result of long-term exposure to analgesics, lead, and other environmental toxins. In some patients with ESRD, the underlying cause of kidney failure is unknown.

PATHOPHYSIOLOGY

Renal injury can occur from a variety of diseases (see Table 8-1) that tend to involve a specific nephron segment initially, such as blood vessels, glomeruli, tubules, or interstitium. Ultimately, a process that affects any portion of the nephron or its surrounding interstitium will go on to impair glomerular filtration as well as other functions of that nephron. Normal renal architecture is lost and replaced with collagen. As this occurs, the size of the kidneys generally decreases.

The kidneys generally fail in an organized fashion. Some nephrons become nonfunctional as a result of injury, whereas other nephrons continue to function at greater than normal capacity as if to compensate for the lost nephrons. This organized process of kidney organ failure is known as the *intact nephron hypothesis* and provides a useful framework for understanding many aspects of CRF. The intact nephrons maintain fluid and solute homeostasis until some irreducible number of functioning nephrons remain. At this point, the patient will develop uremia, and death will occur in weeks to months unless dialysis or transplantation is performed. The intact nephrons adapt to the loss of diseased nephrons by increasing their size, single-nephron GFR (SNGFR), and solute excretion. Increased SNGFR (i.e., hyperfiltration) occurs by dilatation of afferent glomerular arterioles, resulting in enhanced single-nephron plasma flow (Fig. 8-1). Filtration may also be enhanced by increased efferent arteriolar tone. Increased single-nephron plasma flow and SNGFR in remnant nephrons appears to be an adaptive short-term response designed to compensate for the loss of other nephrons. However, the increase in plasma flow and GFR in the surviving nephrons results in an increase in glomerular hydrostatic pressure, which may be maladaptive in the long term.

Chronic renal failure is often progressive even if the inciting cause of injury is removed. The rate of progression varies depending on the individual. The same renal disease may progress to end-stage rapidly in one person (e.g., 1 year) and quite slowly in another (e.g., 10 years). The rate of progression of CRF can be monitored clinically by tracking the reciprocal of serum creatinine over time (described below). A major effort has been mounted to learn the reasons for progression of renal disease and methods for halting or slowing the progression.

A popular explanation for the progressive nature of CRF is termed the *hyperfiltration hypothesis*. The hyperfiltration hypothesis states that the intact nephrons are eventually injured by the increased plasma flow and hydrostatic pressure. Healthy remnant nephrons sustain damage as a result of long-term exposure to increased capillary pressure and flow (see Fig. 8-1). Hyperfiltration injury leads to a characteristic glomerular injury pattern known as focal glomerular sclerosis. This hypothesis potentially explains why renal failure continues to progress even when the initial renal insult is self-limited (e.g., some forms of glomerulonephritis).

Hyperfiltration injury can be diminished by reducing glomerular hydrostatic pressure. Several methods of lowering glomerular pressure have been tried in an effort to slow or halt the progression of CRF. *Antihypertensive therapy* appears to slow the progression of CRF in hypertensive patients. Most agents selectively dilate the afferent arteriole, resulting in increased flow into the glomerular capillaries. At the same time there is a reduction in glomerular capillary pressure as a result of the fall in systemic pressure (see Fig. 8-1). These two processes partially offset each other, yet the net effect of antihypertensive treatment is to slow the rate of CRF progression. Angiotensin converting enzyme inhibitors (ACE inhibitors) are a specific class of antihypertensive drugs that block the conversion of angiotensin I to angiotensin II (AII) within the kidney. AII is a vasoconstrictor but is relatively more selective for the efferent arteriole. By blocking AII formation, ACE inhibitors dilate efferent arterioles more than afferent arterioles (see Fig. 8-1). This selective vasodilation results in a reduction in glomerular capillary pressure and a reduction in hemodynamic injury to the capillary wall. ACE inhibitors slow or prevent the progression of renal failure in experimental animals. Recent studies in humans confirm this selective advantage of ACE inhibitors. Dietary protein restriction may also prevent hyperfiltration injury by lowering the blood flow rate and glomerular capillary pressure in remnant nephrons. Despite much investigation, the required degree of protein restriction and the specific role of this type of intervention have not been fully determined.

Other mechanisms have been proposed to explain the progressive nature of renal failure in addition to hyperfiltration injury. For example, coagulation abnormalities, lipid deposition, and mesangial trapping of macromolecules may lead to progressive damage of intact nephrons.

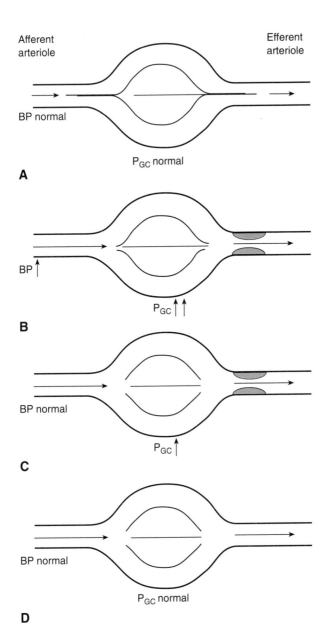

Figure 8-1. Glomerular hemodynamic patterns in the normal state and with chronic renal failure (CRF). (**A**) In the normal state, the systemic blood pressure (BP), afferent arteriolar tone, efferent arteriolar tone, and glomerular capillary pressure (P_{GC}) are all normal. (**B**) In CRF, P_{GC} is elevated in the remaining intact nephrons as a result of increased systemic BP, afferent arteriolar dilation, and efferent arteriolar vasoconstriction. Efferent vasoconstriction is mediated by local release of angiotensin II. (**C**) In CRF, P_{GC} falls if systemic BP is treated with antihypertensive therapy. (**D**) In CRF, P_{GC} falls further if BP is treated with an angiotensin converting enzyme (ACE inhibitor). The ACE inhibitor lowers P_{GC} by selective efferent arteriolar dilation in addition to lowering systemic BP.

METABOLIC CONSEQUENCES OF RENAL FAILURE

Because of a large reserve capacity and compensatory changes in intact nephrons, most individuals can lose at least 90% of glomerular filtration before developing overt clinical signs and symptoms of kidney failure. However, a number of physiochemical changes occur, and patients with renal failure are vulnerable to extreme changes in environmental conditions, which require renal reserve capacity. This section describes the physiologic and biochemical manifestations of CRF, and the following section describes the clinical signs and symptoms that become apparent as GFR falls below approximately 10 ml/minute.

SODIUM HANDLING

CRF is a state in which a diminished number of nephrons are performing at increased capacity to maintain extracellular homeostasis. However, the compensatory efforts of the intact nephrons may not be sufficient for every situation. Patients with CRF have a smaller than normal capacity to excrete a salt load (Figure 8-2). If salt intake exceeds the sodium excretory capacity of the remaining nephrons, a state of excessive sodium accumulation will ensue. Sodium retention results in expansion of the extracellular space, which is manifest as edema and hypertension. Therefore, most patients with CRF will require a sodium-restricted diet as their disease advances.

The ability to conserve sodium also may be compromised in patients with CRF. In rare cases, if sodium intake is excessively low, salt excretion can exceed salt intake, and the patient will develop signs of volume depletion such as low blood pressure and lightheadedness.

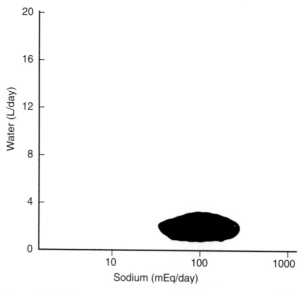

Figure 8-2. Patients with chronic renal failure are unable to handle extreme intake levels of both salt and water. Normal individuals can handle much greater extremes of sodium and water intake than can persons with chronic renal failure. The shaded area denotes theoretical limits for salt and water intake compatible with salt and water balance in a patient with severe chronic renal failure. Salt excess causes edema and hypertension, whereas low salt intake may cause hypovolemia. Water excess may cause hyponatremia, whereas inadequate water intake may cause hypernatremia. (Adapted from Brenner BM, Rector FC, eds. The kidney. 4th ed. Philadelphia: WB Saunders, 1991.)

WATER HANDLING

With advancing CRF, the ability of the kidneys to make urine that is either very dilute or very concentrated becomes compromised (see Fig. 8-2). A dilute urine is required to handle a large water load (see Chap. 1). CRF patients may develop hyponatremia if they drink excessive amounts of water. A concentrated urine is necessary to maximally conserve water under conditions of water deprivation. Inability to maximally conserve water leads to the development of hypernatremia. Patients with CRF are at risk of developing hyponatremia if they drink too much water or hypernatremia if they drink too little water. Fortunately, these manifestations of abnormal water handling seldom occur at usual levels of water intake.

POTASSIUM HANDLING

The ability to excrete potassium is dependent on GFR and distal nephron function. As these become compromised, potassium is retained, and the patient may develop hyperkalemia. This is a serious complication of renal failure because of the risk of fatal arrhythmias and often is an indication for initiation of dialysis. With advanced renal failure, the gut (especially the colon) becomes an important site of potassium secretion. Patients with CRF are advised to restrict potassium intake.

ACID–BASE STATUS

Excretion of the daily acid load depends on excretion of ammonia by the nephron. Although ammonia secretion is increased in intact nephrons, the overall quantity of ammonia excreted is reduced. Hydrogen ion accumulates in the body, resulting in metabolic acidosis (Fig. 8-3). The acidosis is partially buffered by bone, which is a factor in the development of bone disease in patients with renal failure.

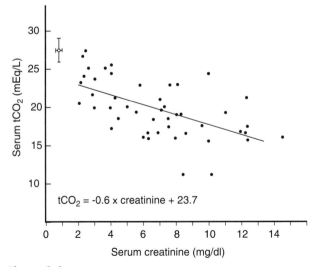

$$tCO_2 = -0.6 \times creatinine + 23.7$$

Figure 8-3. Patients develop metabolic acidosis with progressive loss of glomerular filtration rate. Metabolic acidosis is indicated by a fall in the serum bicarbonate concentration (i.e., total CO_2). (Adapted from Widmer B, Gerhardt RE, Harrington JT, and Cohen JJ. Serum electrolyte and acid base composition. The influence of graded degrees of chronic renal failure. Arch Int Med 1979;39:1099.)

In more advanced stages of CRF, retention of acidic sulfates and phosphates leads to an increase in unmeasured anions (i.e., anion gap acidosis). Patients with CRF often require alkali therapy to neutralize the retained acid load. As the metabolic acidosis becomes severe, dialysis may be required for satisfactory management.

MINERAL METABOLISM

A complex set of alterations in mineral metabolism occurs in CRF, ultimately leading to metabolic bone disease (i.e., renal osteodystrophy) and other toxic manifestations (Fig. 8-4). Renal production of calcitriol, the active form of vitamin D [$1,25(OH)_2D$]), declines as viable renal tissue is lost. With moderate-to-advanced renal failure, the production rate and serum concentration of calcitriol are inadequate to maintain calcium balance, and the patient develops hypocalcemia. Furthermore, the filtration and excretion of inorganic phosphate (PO_4) are decreased in CRF, leading to the development of hyperphosphatemia. As the serum phosphate concentration rises, phosphate and calcium in the plasma form a salt by mass action and precipitate out of the circulation into soft tissue. The resultant loss of calcium further contributes to the hypocalcemia of renal failure. Phosphorus accumulation also directly suppresses calcitriol production, further compounding the problem. The secretion of parathyroid hormone (PTH) is stimulated by the low calcium and calcitriol concentrations. This is a secondary form of hyperparathyroidism in response to known stimuli. In the short term, the secondary hyperparathyroidism of renal failure appears to be a homeostatic mechanism designed to restore the plasma calcium and calcitriol concentrations to normal and repair calcium balance. However, because the underlying problem (i.e., renal failure) remains, hyperparathyroidism is harmful in the long term; it contributes to the musculoskeletal disease of renal failure and is thought to exert other toxic effects as well.

DRUG HANDLING

Drugs that are normally removed by the kidneys will accumulate in patients with renal failure, leading to exaggerated actions and side effects. It is necessary to reduce the dose or extend the dosing interval of drugs that are excreted by the kid-

Figure 8-4. Alterations in mineral metabolism in patients with chronic renal failure are characterized by low calcitriol levels, hyperphosphatemia, hypocalcemia, and secondary hyperparathyroidism. Exogenous intake of aluminum, either in antacids used to bind dietary phosphate or in dialysate fluid, can lead to aluminum intoxication. Renal osteodystrophy encompasses osteitis fibrosa cystica, which is caused by hyperparathyroidism, and osteomalacia, which is caused predominantly by aluminum accumulation in bone. (PTH, parathyroid hormone.)

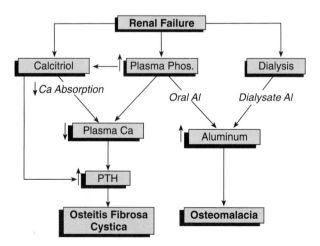

neys. Drugs that are removed by the kidney include aminoglycoside antibiotics, vancomycin, many penicillins, digoxin, and allopurinol. In contrast, drugs such as erythromycin, narcotics, anticoagulants, and phenytoin are removed by the liver and do not require dosage adjustments in renal failure patients. The extracellular protein-binding characteristics of some drugs are changed in renal failure patients. For example, phenytoin is less avidly bound to plasma albumin, and lower total drug concentrations are required for therapeutic effectiveness.

RENAL ENDOCRINE FUNCTION

The production and serum concentration of hormones that are made in the kidney are decreased with CRF. Specifically, calcitriol production is diminished, leading to hypocalcemia and hyperparathyroidism. Also, erythropoietin production declines in CRF, leading to a normochromic, normocytic anemia (Fig. 8-5).

CASE 1

A 33-year-old man has chronic renal failure as a result of polycystic kidney disease. The patient's father and an older sister also have kidney disease, whereas his mother and two other siblings are unaffected. The patient feels well and is employed as a mechanic. Physical examination is significant for a blood pressure of 170/95 mm Hg and bilaterally large, palpable kidneys.

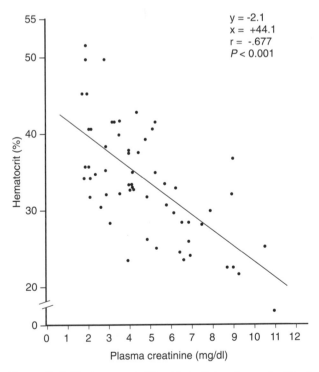

$$y = -2.1$$
$$x = +44.1$$
$$r = -.677$$
$$P < 0.001$$

Figure 8-5. The hematocrit falls with declining glomerular filtration rate in patients with chronic renal failure. Patients develop a normochromic, normocytic anemia, primarily as a result of loss of erythropoietin production by the kidneys. (From McGonigle RJS, Wallin JD, Shadduck RK, and Fisher JW. Erythropoietin deficiency and inhibition of erythropoiesis in renal insufficiency. Kidney Int 1984; 25:437.)

Laboratory evaluation reveals the following serum measurements: urea nitrogen, 88 mg/dl; creatinine, 7.2 mg/dl; sodium, 140 mEq/L; potassium, 6 mEq/L; chloride, 104 mEq/L; bicarbonate, 19 mEq/L; calcium, 8.3 mg/dl; and phosphorus, 6.5 mg/dl.

How do the terms azotemia, uremia, or chronic renal failure apply to this patient? Identify each laboratory alteration present in this patient and explain its pathogenesis.

CASE DISCUSSION

The patient has azotemia, as indicated by elevated levels of serum urea nitrogen and creatinine. However, the patient is not uremic, because he lacks symptoms and signs of kidney failure. He does have chronic renal failure as a result of genetic kidney disease, which has resulted in irreversible damage to normal kidney architecture. Although patients with CRF usually have small, scarred kidneys, those with polycystic disease have large kidneys because of dilation of individual tubules.

This patient has many of the typical laboratory abnormalities that are seen with CRF. The specific abnormalities include the following:

Hyperkalemia. Potassium excretion is impaired because secretion of potassium in the distal nephron is dependent on a high GFR. The ability to excrete a potassium load falls as the GFR falls. Hyperkalemia can be compounded by a high potassium intake and certain medications.

Metabolic acidosis. Acidosis is indicated by the low serum bicarbonate concentration. Acidosis develops with renal failure because of retained organic acids and decreased secretion of ammonia, which is needed for hydrogen ion excretion.

Hypocalcemia. The serum calcium concentration is low in part because of decreased intestinal calcium absorption. Calcium absorption is low because of decreased renal production of calcitriol.

Hyperphosphatemia. Renal excretion of phosphate (PO_4) declines as the GFR falls, leading to hyperphosphatemia.

CLINICAL CONSEQUENCES OF CHRONIC RENAL FAILURE

Virtually every organ system and body function can be affected by renal failure. The earliest symptoms of uremia are usually fatigue, disrupted sleep pattern, decreased appetite, nausea, and vomiting. Uremic manifestations are the result of accumulated toxins (identities unknown for the most part) and disrupted excretory and hormonal function. A systemic listing of uremic manifestations follows, although all of these features are not necessarily seen in every patient.

NEUROLOGIC CONSEQUENCES

The accumulation of uremic toxins affects central nervous system function. The seizure threshold is reduced, manifested initially as asterixis but with the potential of progressing to overt seizures. Mental function can be affected. Initially, this may be seen as subtle electroencephalogram changes, but eventually, patients can develop depressed sensorium. Long-standing CRF also affects the peripheral nervous system in the form of a peripheral sensory neuropathy.

HEMATOLOGIC CONSEQUENCES

Patients are characteristically anemic as a result of deficient production of erythropoietin by the diseased kidneys (see Fig. 8-5). The anemia is normochromic and normocytic and can be largely corrected by administration of exogenous erythropoietin. Platelet number is normal, but function is impaired because of uremic toxins. As a result, patients have a bleeding diathesis. The number of white blood cells is normal, but some studies suggest that immunologic and phagocytic function is impaired by the uremic state, disposing the patients to an increased risk of developing infections.

CARDIOVASCULAR CONSEQUENCES

Most patients with CRF have hypertension. In some cases, the hypertension precedes the onset of kidney injury and may have caused or exacerbated the kidney failure. In other cases, hypertension is clearly secondary to another underlying kidney disease. Sometimes, it is not possible to distinguish which condition occurred first. Hypertension arises from sodium and fluid retention (i.e., volume overload) and release of vasoconstrictive substances such as renin into the circulation. Appropriate therapy consists of controlling the extracellular volume with diuretics or dialysis and vasodilation. CRF patients also have dyslipidemias and, perhaps, a predisposition for atherogenesis. Because of this multitude of cardiovascular risk factors, patients with CRF have a high risk of developing cardiovascular diseases such as myocardial infarction and stroke.

The ability to eliminate a salt load may become compromised in some patients with CRF, leading to expansion of the extracellular volume and edema formation. Congestive heart failure and pulmonary edema may develop, particularly in patients with some degree of underlying heart disease.

With advanced renal failure, patients may develop an acute pericarditis, which appears to be an inflammatory and hemorrhagic response to accumulated uremic toxins in the pericardial space. When this serious complication develops, patients may present with chest pain, shortness of breath, and a pericardial friction rub. Tamponade may ensue, with hypotension and circulatory collapse. Dialysis therapy, by removing the offending toxins, often helps to resolve the problem, although additional therapy is sometimes needed.

SKELETAL MANIFESTATIONS

After an extended period in an environmental milieu characterized by poor calcium absorption and hypocalcemia, hyperparathyroidism, and metabolic acidosis (bone buffers the H^+ ion by releasing calcium), the bones of patients with renal failure tend to degenerate, a process known as renal osteodystrophy (see Fig. 8-4). Bone development may be delayed in children with CRF, contributing to growth retardation. Adult patients may develop bone pain and fractures.

Histologically, the most common bone lesion seen in patients with renal failure is *osteitis fibrosa cystica*, which is caused by PTH excess. The high concentration of PTH stimulates bone turnover by osteoclasts and osteoblasts. The rate of mineral removal exceeds the rate of new mineralization, resulting in increased osteoid, the soft tissue bone matrix. The other major histologic pattern of bone disease in patients with CRF is *osteomalacia*. This pattern is characterized by low bone turnover and decreased bone mineralization. The major cause of osteomalacia in renal failure patients is aluminum intoxication. Aluminum intoxication is an unfortunate iatrogenic problem that occurs in CRF patients who take aluminum antacids over extended periods of time, usually to bind dietary phosphate. Classically, osteomalacia is the lesion of vitamin D deficiency. However, even though patients with renal failure are deficient in the active vitamin D metabolite calcitriol, most patients do not develop osteomalacia unless they have aluminum overload. Every effort is made to minimize aluminum exposure in CRF patients, but it remains a problem.

Soft tissue calcification often occurs in CRF patients as a consequence of severe, poorly controlled hyperphosphatemia. Calcium phosphate precipitates out of the circulation and deposits in soft tissues such as skin, heart, joints, tendons, muscles, and blood vessels, and in other locations. A protean but predictable range of problems arise, including pruritus, cardiac arrhythmias, arthritis, muscle weakness, and peripheral ischemia. These problems may present earlier than and often overshadow the bone disease of renal failure.

GASTROINTESTINAL CONSEQUENCES

Nausea and vomiting are among the earliest symptoms of uremia and can presage anorexia and weight loss. Mucosal inflammation and hemorrhage can occur with advanced renal failure. Patients with uremia have an increased risk of gastrointestinal bleeding because of the formation of arteriovenous malformations in the colon combined with a defect in platelet function.

METABOLIC AND ENDOCRINE CONSEQUENCES

A variety of metabolic abnormalities can be seen in patients with CRF, independent of the diseases that caused the kidney failure in the first place. Potential problems include glucose intolerance and insulin resistance, hyperlipidemia, and decreased levels of testosterone and estrogen. Fertility is markedly diminished in women with CRF.

CASE 2

A 65-year-old woman has CRF as a result of chronic glomerulonephritis. Three months ago she felt well; her BUN was 70 mg/dl, and her creatinine was 7.5 mg/dl. She now returns to your office complaining of anorexia, vomiting, and malaise. On further questioning, you learn that she also has pruritus, difficulty sleeping at night, and pleuritic chest pain. Physical examination reveals a blood pressure of 146/92 mm Hg, a pericardial friction rub, and bilateral ankle edema. What do you think accounts for this change in her condition over 3 months? Are these changes unexpected? What is the cause of her symptoms? Does this patient have uremia? What should be done?

CASE DISCUSSION

The most likely explanation is that there has been further deterioration of her renal function, which was already marginal 3 months earlier. This is not unexpected, because CRF is often progressive.

She has typical signs and symptoms of advanced uremia. The anorexia and vomiting are common gastrointestinal manifestations of uremia. Malaise and fatigue are the result of renal failure and anemia caused by deficient renal erythropoietin production. Sleep disturbance is an early neurologic symptom; she likely has other subtle central nervous system problems with concentration and memory. Pruritus often occurs as the serum phosphorus concentration increases. The resultant increase in the serum calcium phosphate product leads to precipitation in soft tissues such as skin. Itching is a consequence of local irritation from the calcium phosphate deposits. The pleuritic chest pain and friction rub are the result of pericarditis. Pericarditis occurs because of irritation of the pericardial membrane by unrecognized uremic toxins. This is a worrisome development because of the possibility of progression to pericardial tamponade and hypotension.

She does indeed have advanced symptoms of uremia. Dialysis should be initiated immediately. Evaluation should be undertaken to rule out pericardial tamponade. From this point on, this woman will require regular dialysis treatments.

MANAGEMENT OF CHRONIC RENAL FAILURE

DISEASE-SPECIFIC THERAPY

Specific treatment should be undertaken to arrest the progression of renal diseases that have the potential to cause scarring and irreversible renal failure. Specific therapies are available for certain inflammatory diseases, such as systemic lupus erythematosus, vasculitis, and some forms of glomerulonephritis. Evidence indicates that aggressive treatment of diabetes and hypertension will lower the chance of kidney damage.

TREATMENT OF HYPERTENSION

Control of blood pressure appears to be beneficial for all hypertensive patients with kidney failure. A reduction in systemic pressure causes a commensurate fall in glomerular capillary pressure and hyperfiltration forces that can cause progressive kidney failure. Any agent or maneuver that lowers blood pressure appears to be helpful, but ACE inhibitors may confer added protection by selectively lowering resistance of the efferent glomerular arterioles and decompressing the capillaries even more than agents that selectively dilate the afferent arteriole bed.

DIET

A low-protein diet appears to decrease glomerular capillary pressure and may slow the progression of renal failure. Restriction of dietary protein intake to 40 to 60 g/day is often recommended for patients with CRF who are not protein malnourished. Patients with advanced renal failure also should be restricted in the intake of potassium and sodium because of the tendency to develop hyperkalemia and volume overload, respectively. Water restriction may also be necessary in patients who are prone to the development of hyponatremia. Dietary phosphate should be restricted to avoid hyperphosphatemia.

DIURETICS FOR EDEMA

Edema occurs frequently in patients with CRF because of the limited ability of the diseased kidney to excrete a salt load. In patients with nephrotic syndrome, edema may also develop because of a low serum albumin concentration; albumin is the source of oncotic pressure that determines the amount of fluid held in the vascular compartment. Peripheral edema is uncomfortable, induces strain on the heart, and often contributes to systemic hypertension. Pulmonary edema causes dyspnea and respiratory failure. Edema should be treated with dietary salt restriction and diuretics. A realistic level of salt restriction for ambulatory patients is 2 g/day of sodium (88 mEq/day). Patients with a creatinine concentration above approximately 2 mg/dl do not respond to thiazide diuretics and should receive a loop diuretic such as furosemide, bumetanide, or ethycrynic acid.

PREVENTION AND TREATMENT OF RENAL OSTEODYSTROPHY

Several measures are employed to prevent and treat the mineral and bone abnormalities of CRF. Patients should be placed on a diet low in phosphorus to abrogate hyperphosphatemia. Phosphate binding agents should be given with meals to decrease phosphate absorption. Calcium salts are preferred for this purpose, because they not only bind dietary phosphate but also provide needed supplemental calcium. Aluminum gels were routinely used in the past for binding phosphate, but some patients developed aluminum intoxication over many years of exposure, and these agents should be avoided if possible. The active form of vitamin D, $1,25(OH)_2D$ or calcitriol, can be given to increase calcium absorption and to directly suppress PTH secretion. The goal of preventive therapy is to correct the hyperphosphatemia and hypocalcemia without causing aluminum intoxication. Bone health is likely to be maintained if these goals are met. For established bone disease, additional measures may be necessary, including parathyroidectomy.

VIGILANT MONITORING OF ALL DRUGS

Renally excreted drugs will accumulate in patients with decreased GFR. Therefore, it is important to lower the dose or extend the dosing interval when these drugs are used in patients with CRF. Drugs that are eliminated by the liver do not generally require dose adjustments in CRF patients.

END-STAGE RENAL DISEASE MANAGEMENT

RENAL REPLACEMENT THERAPY

The measures described previously should be employed as needed in patients with progressive CRF. Many patients can exist in a symptom-free state until the

GFR falls below approximately 10 ml/minute. At lower GFR levels, patients reliably develop clinical manifestations of renal failure, such as hyperkalemia, metabolic acidosis, fluid overload, and the signs and symptoms of uremia (i.e., vomiting, pruritus, sleep disturbances, pericarditis, asterixis, and seizures). At this stage (i.e., ESRD), it becomes imperative to provide renal replacement therapy, or the patient will die of mounting complications. Renal replacement therapy consists of dialysis or tranplantation. Two major forms of dialysis are available: hemodialysis and peritoneal dialysis.

HEMODIALYSIS

For hemodialysis, a vascular fistula or graft is surgically placed in an extremity to allow access to the blood circulation using special needles connected to sterile tubing (Fig. 8-6). A dialysis machine based on a roller pump is used to withdraw blood from the patient at a high flow rate (i.e., >250 ml/minute). The blood is routed though a special dialyzer, which is a semipermeable membrane across which fluid and uremic toxins can cross. A dialysate fluid is run on the other side of the membrane to promote diffusive exchange of solutes. After passing though the dialyzer, the purified blood is returned to the patient. Typically, hemodialysis is performed for 4 hours three times per week.

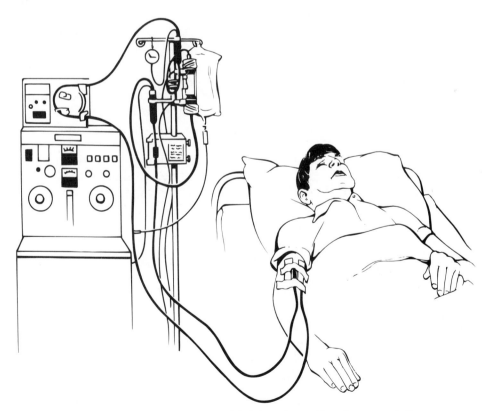

Figure 8-6. Apparatus used to perform hemodialysis in patients with end-stage renal disease.

PERITONEAL DIALYSIS

Peritoneal dialysis uses the semipermeable peritoneal cavity for fluid and solute exchange (Fig. 8-7). A sterile Silastic catheter is routed from the peritoneal cavity through a subcutaneous tunnel to an exit site on the abdominal wall. Sterile dialysis fluid is run into the peritoneal cavity and allowed to equilibrate with the patient's extracellular fluid compartment. The equilibrated dialysate containing waste products and fluid is then drained and discarded. This procedure can usually be done by the patient at home and avoids the inconvenience of frequent visits to a center for scheduled dialysis treatments. Several variations of this technique are available; the most common is continuous ambulatory peritoneal dialysis (CAPD), in which the patient performs four exchanges of approximately 2 L spaced equally throughout the day.

TRANSPLANTATION

Kidney transplantation has become a routine treatment for ESRD and, for many patients, provides the most physiologic and well-tolerated form of renal replacement therapy. Organs are obtained from cadavers, living relatives, or increasingly, from living nonrelatives. Cadaver kidneys are obtained from victims of sudden death, provided the organ is removed prior to discontinuation of life support. Living donors generally do very well with a single kidney. The donor organ is transplanted into the ESRD patient in the iliac fossa with vascular anastomoses to the

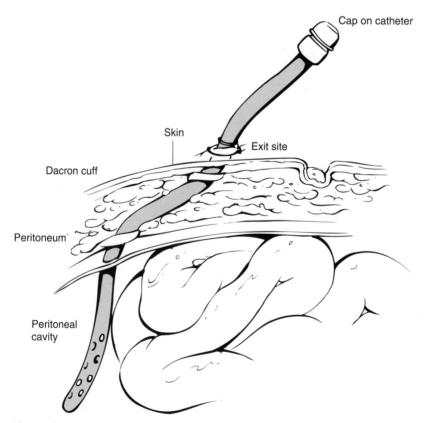

Figure 8-7. Peritoneal dialysis set-up for patients with end-stage renal disease.

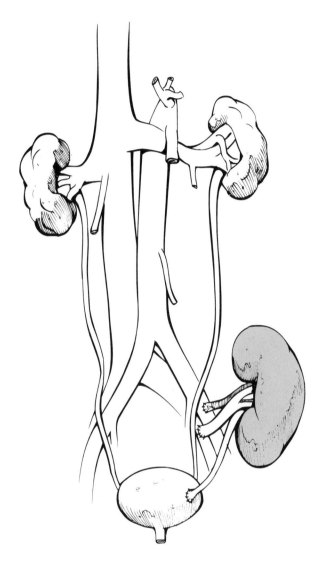

Figure 8-8. Transplanted kidneys are generally placed in the iliac fossa of the recipient. The iliac vessels are used for vascular supply to and from the transplanted kidneys (i.e., allograft). The allograft ureter is attached to the recipient's bladder.

iliac vessels (Fig. 8-8). Extensive tissue typing and testing for preformed antibodies must be done to prevent immunologic rejection of the transplanted organ. Furthermore, patients must be treated prophylactically with immunosuppressive agents to lower the risk of acute rejection. The most common agents in use are corticosteroids, cyclosporine, and azathioprine. Several polyclonal and monoclonal antibody preparations directed against lymphocytes are also used to prevent or treat rejection. In addition to rejection, transplant patients have an enhanced risk of developing opportunistic infections and neoplasms. Nonetheless, the 1-year survival rate for cadaver kidney transplants is in the range of 80%.

METHOD FOR TRACKING THE PROGRESSION OF CHRONIC KIDNEY DISEASE

Once the kidneys have sustained a substantial degree of damage, progressive deterioration of kidney function over time can often be expected. Progression may occur because of an ongoing disease process, such as diabetes, or because of the deleterious effects of glomerular hypertension within intact nephrons. When renal failure is progressive, the GFR tends to decline in a linear fashion over time (Fig. 8-9). This empirical observation can be used to infer superimposed changes in renal status and to predict the time to ESRD (i.e., when dialysis treatment will be necessary). In clinical practice, the serial measurement of GFR or even creatinine clearance is difficult and fraught with inaccuracies. Fortunately, the reciprocal of the plasma creatinine concentration can be used instead of GFR or creatinine clearance to estimate the rate of progression. Recall that creatinine clearance provides a reasonable estimate of GFR:

$$GFR \approx \text{creatinine clearance} = \frac{U_{Cr}V}{P_{Cr}}$$

where U_{Cr} is the urine creatinine concentration, V is the urine flow rate, and P_{Cr} is the plasma creatinine concentration. Creatinine is a breakdown product of skeletal

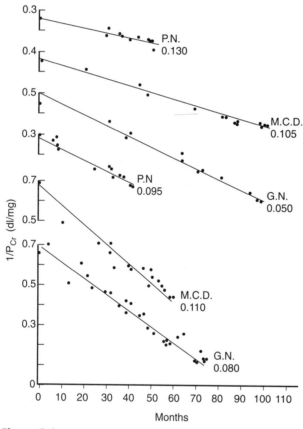

Figure 8-9. The reciprocal of plasma creatinine $(1/P_{Cr})$ tends to fall linearly over time in patients with progressive renal failure, regardless of the underlying etiology. The rate of progression varies greatly among different patients (i.e., G.N., M.C.D., and P.N.). (Adapted from Mitch WE, Walser M, Buffington GA, Lemann J Jr. A simple method of estimating progression of chronic renal failure. Lancet 1976;1:1326.)

muscle. If body muscle mass is stable, then the production and excretion rates of creatinine per unit time (i.e., $U_{Cr}V$) will be relatively constant. The equation thus can be written as follows:

$$GFR \approx creatinine\ clearance = \frac{U_{Cr}V}{P_{Cr}} = \frac{constant}{P_{Cr}} \propto \frac{1}{P_{Cr}}$$

by which it follows that the reciprocal of plasma creatinine ($1/P_{Cr}$) can be used to track changes in GFR (Fig. 8-10).

Changes in the slope of $1/P_{Cr}$ versus time can be used to indicate a change in the rate of progression of renal failure. A steeper slope indicates that progression is more rapid than expected, perhaps because of a superimposed insult such as pyelonephritis or renal vein thrombosis. A shallower slope indicates slower-than-expected progression; this is the goal of antihypertensive and dietary therapy. For most individuals, the indications for initiation of dialysis will be met by the time the plasma creatinine reaches 10 mg/dl or the reciprocal plasma creatinine reaches 0.1. For a patient with a known rate of progression, the approximate time until dialysis is necessary can be crudely estimated by extrapolation of the $1/P_{Cr}$-versus-time relation. The assumption of a linear decline in $1/P_{Cr}$ over time has been challenged, but the technique is often useful if its limitations are appreciated.

CASE 3

A 62-year-old man has long-standing type II (i.e., adult onset, nonketosis prone) diabetes complicated by retinopathy and a peripheral sensory neuropathy. Two years ago, his serum creatinine was 1.0 mg/dl (i.e., normal), but there was 3+ protein on urine dipstick and 6.8 g of protein/24-hour urine collection. At subsequent 6-month visits, the serum creatinine concentration was 1.2, 1.3, 1.9, and 2.3 mg/dl. The patient was referred to you and, recognizing the steady deterioration of renal function, you start the patient on a low-protein diet and an ACE inhibitor to control blood pressure. At subsequent 6-month check-ups, the serum creatinine is 2.6, 2.8, 3.1, and 3.5 mg/dl.

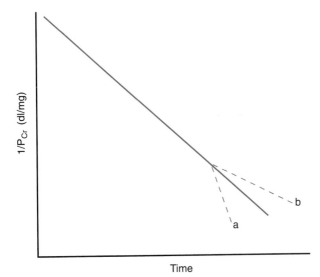

Figure 8-10. Changes in the slope of the reciprocal of plasma creatinine ($1/P_{Cr}$) versus time can indicate superimposed effects of factors that accelerate (curve a) or slow (curve b) the progression of chronic renal failure. Time to end-stage renal disease can be estimated by extrapolation of $1/P_{Cr}$.

Plot reciprocal serum creatinine ($1/P_{Cr}$) versus time for this patient. Describe the slope. Did your therapy appear to change the course of the kidney failure? If you assume that this patient will have to start dialysis treatment when the serum creatinine reaches 8 mg/dl, estimate how long until this happens. How do the treatments you started influence the progression of the kidney disease? What do you think is the cause of this patient's kidney failure and why?

CASE DISCUSSION

Reciprocal serum creatinine fell in an approximately linear fashion for the first 2 years. After the blood pressure and dietary treatment were instituted, the slope flattened, indicating that the rate of renal function loss was decreased. Dialysis will be required for this patient when the serum creatinine reaches 8 mg/dl, corresponding to a reciprocal creatinine of 0.13 dl/mg. This would have occurred at approximately 3 years without treatment, and appears to have been prolonged to 6.5 years with the institution of treatment (Fig. 8-11).

The exact mechanisms are not definitively known; however, it appears that treating high blood pressure extends kidney life by reducing hydraulic pressure within the intact glomerular capillaries. ACE inhibitors selectively dilate the efferent arteriole, leading to an even greater reduction in glomerular capillary pressure. High protein intake causes an increase in GFR and glomerular capillary pressure; these changes are diminished with a low-protein diet.

This patient most likely has chronic renal failure as a result of diabetes. The diagnosis of diabetic nephropathy is supported by the history of long-

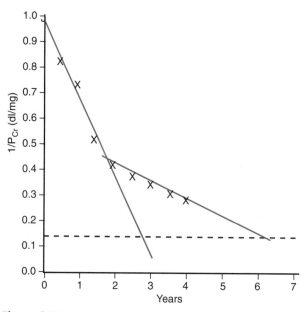

Figure 8-11.

standing diabetes, the presence of other diabetic complications (i.e., retinopathy and neuropathy), and proteinuria that preceded the development of kidney failure. Diabetes is the most common cause of CRF and ESRD.

SELECTED READING

Brenner BM, Meyer TW, Hostetter TH. Dietary protein intake and the progressive nature of kidney disease. N Engl J Med 1982;307:652.

Eschbach JW, Egrie JC, Downing MR, Browne JK, Adamson JW. Correction of the anemia of end-stage renal disease with recombinant human erythropoietin. N Engl J Med 1987;316:73.

Fine LG. The uremic syndrome: adaptive mechanisms and therapy. Hosp Pract 1987;Sept:59.

Kurtzman NA. Chronic renal failure: metabolic and clinical consequences. Hosp Pract 1982;Aug:107.

Lee DBN, Goodman WG, Coburn JW. Renal osteodystrophy: some new questions on an old disorder. Am J Kidney Dis 1988;5:365.

Mitch WE, Walser M, Buffington GA, Lemann J Jr. A simple method of estimating progression of chronic renal failure. Lancet 1976;1:1326.

Page numbers followed by *t* or *f* indicate tables or figures, respectively.

177